Coping Successfully

Coping Successfully with Hepatitis C

Richard English
and
Dr Graham Foster

Robinson
LONDON

Robinson Publishing Ltd
7 Kensington Church Court
London W8 4SP

This revised edition first published 1999

First published by Robinson Publishing Ltd 1997

A copy of the British Library Cataloguing in Publication Data
for this title is available from the British Library.

ISBN 1–84119–070–5

Important Note
This book is not intended to be a substitute for medical advice or
treatment. Any person with a condition requiring medical attention
should consult a qualified medical practitioner or suitable therapist.

Printed and bound in EC

Contents

Hugh, a 40-year-old patient with cirrhosis, offers hope:

'Although news of having chronic hepatitis C infection plunged me into darkness, I've found faith in adversity. I'm learning to help myself by asking others for help. Although this seems like a paradox, it works in a way I can't explain. In spite of my reduced quality of life, I'm coping with my illness and flourishing. I've regained my human dignity in the face of grave uncertainty.'

Introduction

The World Health Organization estimates that 170 million people are infected with hepatitis C, of which 3.9 million live in the United States and 400,000 in Britain. The huge cost in medical, social, and human resources has overshadowed the AIDS problem.

The hepatitis C virus is sly and powerful, spreading throughout the world community regardless of age, race, class or religion. The principal groups at risk are recipients of blood products, including haemophiliacs, and past and present intravenous drug users. However, certain southern Italian old-age pensioners, Chinese housewives and Egyptian businessmen have all been diagnosed.

Chronic hepatitis C damages the liver. At its most dangerous, it leads to cirrhosis or primary liver cancer. Some long-term patients die prematurely, while others have reduced quality of life due to end-stage hepatic complications.

The progression of the disease is highly variable. For those with a moderate to severe infection, it may take anything from ten to forty years for the liver to degenerate significantly. A few lucky patients may not experience any deterioration at all.

The advance of medical science in the last few years

marks a shift from panic to limited optimism about the future for many chronic hepatitis C patients. Until recently, the only treatment available was interferon, which has a 15 per cent success rate. Now that interferon is combined with other drugs, most notably with ribavirin, there is a 40 per cent chance of clearing the virus. Those in need of a liver transplant can take comfort from rapidly improving surgical procedures.

This book gives up-to-date information on hepatitis C, its consequences, its prevention and the process of managing chronic illness. It contains the latest research into drug treatments, as well as evaluations of western complementary medicine (WCM) and traditional Chinese medicine (TCM).

The primary purpose of the authors is to set out a programme of action of how patients can learn to live within the limitations imposed by their illness. There is advice on how to maintain work life, eat sensibly, form a moderate exercise plan, join self-help networks and maintain social and family life.

The book also aims to educate carers, whether they are professional or family, friends and partners, by providing a clear and comprehensive account of hepatitis C and its effects. We have drawn upon an immense wealth of experience and hope of people with hepatitis C, who have learned to flourish in spite of their condition. Their voices and inspiration are evident throughout the text.

1

What is Hepatitis C?

The hepatitis C virus (often abbreviated to HCV or, informally, 'hep C') makes its home in the liver, where it replicates and produces new, infectious hepatitis C particles. The virus also spreads to white blood cells and, in very small amounts, circulates in the bloodstream. If it goes unchecked, the virus can injure the liver, in extreme cases to the point of failure. There may be no symptoms at all during the early phases of the condition, even if a process of inexorable destruction is underway.

According to the most recent estimates, it takes at least twenty years for significant liver scarring to develop. However, once the scars become permanent, this vital organ tends to deteriorate at an accelerating pace. Ultimately, a patient may develop end-stage disease or contract liver cancer, both of which are frequently fatal conditions.

Why You Need Your Liver

Your liver is necessary for your health and well-being. It is the largest organ in your body, weighs about three pounds (a little under one and a half kilograms) and is located in the upper right-hand side of the abdomen, where most of it is protected by the ribcage. Its primary tasks are to:

- break down and store food absorbed from the gut;
- detoxify all the poisonous chemicals your body is given, for example, alcohol and drugs;
- store energy by stockpiling sugar;
- manufacture proteins that help the body to be healthy and to grow;
- store iron reserves, vitamins and other minerals;
- make bile to digest your food;
- produce clotting factors in the blood;
- help defend you against the germs present in your body by manufacturing protective proteins.

Very simply, the liver acts both as a battery, storing various essential products, and as a filter, detoxifying certain harmful substances. Without it, you cannot live.

Types of Hepatitis

'Hepatitis' means 'liver inflammation'. There are many kinds of 'viral hepatitis', which is 'liver inflammation due to the presence of a virus'. Viral hepatitis may be acute, fulminant or chronic.

- *Acute hepatitis* is liver inflammation that lasts for less than six months and does not normally cause any long-term problems. It is a fairly mild disease that after a brief period of liver inflammation is completely cured.
- *Fulminant hepatitis* is a severe form of short-term hepatitis in which the liver is rapidly and almost completely destroyed. This condition is rare; it is usually fatal,

although emergency transplantation can sometimes be life-saving.

- *Chronic hepatitis* is liver inflammation that lasts for longer than six months. It may lead to scarring in the liver, and eventually to cirrhosis, which is irreversible scarring.

A virus is an entity so small that it cannot be seen under even a very powerful light microscope. It invades the body through one or more channels. Some, for example, flu or cold viruses, are inhaled. Others, for instance, herpes simplex, enter through the oral and genital tracts.

Several viruses are commonly associated with hepatitis. They do not all infect a patient by the same means, and so they are given different labels, alphabetically from A to G roughly in the order in which they were discovered.

Hepatitis A

Hepatitis A is an acute infection. It is caught after oral ingestion of the virus, usually by drinking or eating water or food contaminated with faeces from an infected person (the virus is excreted from the body in faeces). The virus is not often found in the United Kingdom or America, but is common in some Mediterranean and third world countries. You are most likely to catch it while travelling, on holiday or from someone who has recently arrived from abroad.

You are advised to have an inoculation against this virus if you are going to an area where it is prevalent. If you catch it, you will be ill for several months, experiencing jaundice, tiredness, nausea and depression. The problem eventually clears up, although a tiny number of hepatitis A patients develop fulminant hepatitis.

3

Hepatitis B
Hepatitis B is an acute infection for 90 per cent of infected adults and a chronic infection for 10 per cent. A small proportion of infected adults develop fulminant hepatitis. Hepatitis B is a highly infectious virus and is transmitted sexually and through blood. You can have an inoculation against it.

Those who have the acute infection suffer in much the same way as those with hepatitis A. A small proportion of adults infected with hepatitis B, however, do not develop the typical symptoms of jaundice and malaise: they have a resistant infection that does not resolve and becomes chronic. This chronic hepatitis B infection causes slow, progressive liver damage that often leads to cirrhosis and/or liver cancer. Although chronic infection is uncommon in adults, infection with the hepatitis B virus in childhood most often leads to the chronic form of the illness; transmission of hepatitis B from mothers to their children is responsible for chronic infection in many hundreds of millions of people worldwide.

Hepatitis C
Hepatitis C causes an acute infection in some individuals but leads to a chronic infection in the majority of those who are exposed to it. Of those who have the chronic form of hepatitis C, 30 per cent have a mild and 70 per cent an aggressive form of the disease. In its mild state the disease is likely to cause minor damage to the liver, and the risk of serious complications is small. In the aggressive form, severe destruction of the liver is probable and dangerous symptoms are likely to make themselves felt eventually.

Hepatitis D
Hepatitis D (also known as the delta virus) is only found in patients who are already infected with hepatitis B. It is very

dangerous, as it magnifies the severity of hepatitis B and is virtually untreatable.

Hepatitis E
Hepatitis E is similar to hepatitis A in that it is always an acute infection and spreads through oral/faecal contamination. It is rarely found in Europe or America but is common in Asia, Mexico and Africa, where epidemics may occur. Although acute hepatitis E is typically a mild disease, infection in pregnant women is extremely dangerous and leads to fulminant hepatitis in a high proportion of cases.

Hepatitis F
'Hepatitis F' is actually a misnomer, in that the term does not refer to an identified virus: the original description of hepatitis F has not been confirmed and it seems likely that no such virus exists. This letter has now been dropped from the hepatitis alphabet.

Hepatitis G
Hepatitis G is a recently identified virus that is found throughout the world. Although hepatitis G has been associated with acute and chronic infections, many patients infected with hepatitis G are completely well, with no liver disease.

Most experts believe that hepatitis G is not really a hepatitis virus at all but is simply a benign virus that is carried by many healthy people. A large number of patients infected with HCV are also infected with hepatitis G and it is probable that such dual infection is not of any special significance. The liver disease is due to the HCV and the presence of another virus does not alter the natural history of the original disease process.

HIV and HCV

Whatever else you get wrong, remember that HCV is *not* HIV. HIV is short for 'human immunodeficiency virus'. People infected by HIV inevitably progress to AIDS, which is a fatal condition.

The virus that causes AIDS – HIV is a member of a family of viruses known as 'retroviruses'. HCV is a member of a completely different family of viruses (the 'flaviviruses') that have their own structures, genetic material and effects. There is no significant structural similarity between HIV and HCV.

HIV is much more infectious than HCV and can be transmitted sexually as well as by blood. HIV is especially prevalent among homosexuals, former and current intravenous drug users, and blood recipients. Since HCV is also prevalent in former and current intravenous drug users it is inevitable that a small number of people (especially intravenous drug users) will be infected with both viruses. This does not occur very often, and the vast majority of people who have HCV do not have HIV.

The History of Hepatitis C and its Variants

Hepatitis C was identified in 1989. Prior to its discovery, the condition was known as 'non-A non-B hepatitis'. Many journal articles, medical textbooks and pamphlets written before 1989 refer to non-A non-B hepatitis.

Strictly speaking, HCV is not one virus but a group of closely related viral strains. There are thought to be at least six kinds of HCV, which are called 'genotypes'. The known kinds have been numbered from one upwards, with subtypes a, b and c, in order of discovery. So far the following have been identified: 1a, b and c; 2a and b; 3a; 4a; 5a; 6a.

6

Genotypes 1a, 1b, 2a, 2b and 3a are found principally in blood donors and patients with chronic hepatitis C from countries in western Europe and the United States. Infection with type 1b is commonly found in patients who live around the Mediterranean, while in the rest of Europe, type 3a has infected young people with a history of intravenous drug use. Type 1b accounts for most infections in people aged 50 or over. Type 4a is the most prevalent in Egypt and many other parts of the Middle East and Africa. Type 5a is confined largely to South Africa, while type 6a is found in Hong Kong and Southeast Asia.

If you have hepatitis C, which genotype you have may be significant for purposes of your prognosis and treatment.

Common Symptoms

Many, but by no means all, patients infected with hepatitis C notice symptoms in the early stages of infection. William, a 39-year-old company director from Holland Park, London, says:

'I didn't know what was wrong with me, but I knew that something was amiss. I felt increasingly tired, run down, and depressed. I kept feeling that I was going to be sick. It was as if I had a bad hangover. And yet I hadn't had an alcoholic drink for years . . .

'During the day, I could barely stay awake. In the evenings, I stopped going out and started to go to bed early. I became fussy about my food. In general, I switched from being perky and animated into being irritable and unreasonable. I lost my appetite for life. My sole objective was "to get a good night's sleep". The worrying thing was that even with plenty of rest and healthy food, I soon became lethargic and nauseous again.'

William's description of how he felt brings out the subtle nature of some of the symptoms that may be associated with infection by hepatitis C.

One of the most puzzling features of hepatitis C is that it affects different people in different ways. Some patients with chronic infection have absolutely no symptoms whatsoever, while others are incapacitated by their disease. There is no obvious relationship between how you feel and what is going on in your liver.

The cause of the symptoms associated with hepatitis C is unknown. They may be related to the body's attempts to get rid of the virus, or to infection of the white blood cells. As in William's case, tiredness, nausea and malaise are the most common complaints.

Tiredness

Many (but by no means all) people infected by HCV suffer from tiredness. This is sometimes referred to as 'lassitude' or 'fatigue'. What it amounts to is that you feel permanently drained. Energy levels fall and there seems to be no way of boosting them. If you are an undiagnosed HCV patient, this leads to further anxiety since you cannot understand why you feel so jaded all the time.

It is not yet known why such large numbers of people with HCV feel tired. It is not simply the effects of the virus damaging the liver, since some HCV patients with only mild hepatitis suffer from lassitude. There is no clear correlation between the severity of the liver inflammation and fatigue.

Nausea

Some HCV patients feel sick or nauseous. When you eat a meal, you may often feel queasy directly afterwards. Sometimes just seeing or smelling food may make you feel sick. Fatty foods are particularly likely to bring on nausea. The sensations are similar to low-level but continuous seasickness.

Malaise

A considerable number of patients with chronic HCV complain of malaise. This is a general feeling of ill-health, sometimes thought of as a barely discernible flu. You may find yourself doing fewer of the things you have been used to doing because you feel run down. Like fatigue, malaise can take the form of a lack of energy or a tendency to tire easily. Your capacity for work may diminish, while your need for sleep increases.

Activities that you formerly enjoyed may become too much for you. You may stop going out in the evenings or going away for the weekends, or you may just give up some of your hobbies. The boundaries of your existence will narrow, probably without your noticing or caring.

Malaise is often accompanied by depression, which is experienced as the presence of increasingly black thoughts. You may turn very gradually from an optimist (assuming you were one!) into an inveterate pessimist. You may become progressively irritable and unable to think positively. Formerly, life had seemed full of hope and good experiences; now it has lost its gloss.

Wendy's hepatitis has contaminated her outlook on life so that she has become mentally as well as physically debilitated:

'Since I've had hep C I've become very depressed. Often I can't go out because I feel so ill. For weeks at a time I'm in bed with flu-like symptoms. I can't work any more. I had a career as an actress and was doing very well at it.

'When I feel a bit better I can only do one thing on a day-to-day basis. If I go to see the doctor, that's all I'm fit for. I feel hopeless. What's the point of going on? I get frightened that I could die from this illness.'

Less Common Symptoms

There are other symptoms of which only a minority of hepatitis patients complain. They tend to be mild and sporadic, although a very small proportion of patients find them burdensome.

Headaches and Joint Pains
Some patients have migraine-type headaches, particularly on waking. A small dose of paracetamol is usually all that is needed to relieve the pain.

'Arthralgias', or pains in the joints, may be associated with chronic HCV. It is reassuring that arthralgias associated with this virus do not lead to deformity or destruction of the joints, as with rheumatoid arthritis. Generally, they are felt in the morning as an uncomfortable stiffness in the fingers and toes. As with the headaches, a small dose of paracetamol relieves the symptom.

Diarrhoea, Irritable Bowel and Bladder
The presence of HCV may affect the digestive system, and, very rarely, infection can be associated with diarrhoea. Patients sometimes lament that they have to defecate many times a day and that their stools are loose or liquid.

It is important to remember that there is a large range of causes of diarrhoea, and it is unusual for hepatitis C to cause bowel problems. If you suffer in this way it is recommended that you are thoroughly investigated to ensure that there is no other, potentially treatable, cause of your diarrhoea.

In some cases irritable bowel and bladder syndromes develop. These problems amount to the frequent and urgent need to eliminate, to the extent of causing severe discomfort. They require specialized treatment, about which your liver doctor can advise you.

Cognitive Disturbance

A few patients experience 'cognitive disturbance'. This is a general term referring to interference with the mind's ability to perform its normal functions. An impaired memory or exceptional vagueness are examples of this symptom.

Katherine, 41, a divorcee with two children, finds she suffers disorientation as well as other limitations upon her mental faculties:

> 'My concentration is appalling. My memory is absolutely terrible and quite often I can't find words which I know perfectly well . . . I can't retrieve them. I can't always remember people's names. Sometimes I'm in a room and I don't know why I've gone in there or what I was doing a few moments before.'

Associated Medical Problems

A large number of medical disorders have been associated with HCV infection. Some of these associations are simply coincidence; many patients are infected with HCV and, purely by chance, some of these patients will develop, or already suffer from, other clinical disorders. However, some distressing conditions are regularly found in patients with chronic hepatitis C, and so are probably caused by the virus.

Thyroid Disease

The thyroid gland is a small gland situated in the neck which produces a chemical – a hormone – called thyroxine. Thyroxine has many functions, but the most important is to speed up the body's metabolism to an appropriate basic metabolic rate and keep it there. A deficiency of thyroxine causes pronounced fatigue.

A significant number of patients with HCV develop problems with their thyroid gland leading to a reduction in the production of thyroxine. This can lead to profound tiredness. Pinpointing the reduction in the level of thyroxine as the cause of fatigue is important, since tablets containing thyroxine can be prescribed to correct the deficiency and so diminish the symptoms. Because of this possibility, most liver specialists routinely measure the level of thyroxine in the blood of patients with HCV. This is done by a simple blood test which can be performed on the same blood sample that is used to carry out liver function tests.

You are warned that thyroxine is a dangerous drug. An excess of thyroxine can cause the heart to beat very rapidly and may be fatal. It is essential that you *only* take thyroxine tablets if the level of thyroxine has been found to be low, and that the treatment is carefully monitored by your doctor. You should *never* take thyroxine tablets simply to ease the tiredness that is frequently associated with HCV. Unless thyroxine deficiency has been diagnosed, the drug will not ease your symptoms and may be dangerous.

Other Glandular Disorders
People with chronic HCV may suffer from dry eyes and a dry mouth. Studies of the salivary and lachrymal glands of HCV patients suggest that the virus can infect these organs and may give rise to these unpleasant symptoms.

It is important to let your doctor know if you are suffering from these problems as they can be treated. Dry eyes can be eased by artificial tear preparations, used as eye drops, and artificial salivary sprays can relieve discomfort in the mouth.

Some authorities believe that HCV can also cause inflammation of the pancreas. The pancreas is a large gland situated in the upper part of the abdomen, just behind the stomach. 'Pancreatitis' – inflammation of the pancreas – causes severe upper abdominal pain and vomiting. In addition to HCV, a number of other disorders can cause inflammation of the pancreas. Alcohol abuse and gallstones are the most common causes. Inflammation of the pancreas can be severe and sometimes requires treatment in hospital. In most cases it is mild, although even then it tends to cause constant upper abdominal and back pain. In general, treatment is not very effective, although a variety of drugs can be tried to reduce the distress caused by the condition.

Kidney Disease
A few patients with hepatitis C develop inflammation of the kidney (glomerulonephritis). This complaint does not normally cause symptoms but is detected by special blood and urine tests. Glomerulonephritis caused by HCV requires specialist treatment.

Skin Disease
Chronic infection with hepatitis C can be associated with a number of different skin diseases. These are uncommon and require specialist management. If you notice any unusual spots or blisters on your skin you should tell your doctor so that appropriate tests can be performed and treatment recommended.

Cirrhosis

If your liver remains inflamed long enough, it will sustain irreversible damage. This is called 'cirrhosis'. It is a scarring or hardening of previously normal tissue, which ultimately forms itself into nodules of scar tissue that surround areas of inflamed liver, and is a very real danger for those suffering from chronic hepatitis. It may develop in up to 30 per cent of patients with chronic HCV, although it is most often found in older patients, who have had active hepatitis for twenty years or more.

The liver is a sturdy organ with a powerful capacity to repair itself. In the event of most kinds of damage, the liver is able to replace unhealthy with healthy cells. However, in the case of prolonged inflammation due to the presence of HCV, it cannot replenish itself. At first, small areas of the liver become cirrhotic as isolated pockets of liver cells are wrecked and replaced by scar tissue. Gradually, larger and larger numbers of healthy cells are destroyed and dangerous consequences result. For one thing, blood cannot flow properly through the liver; for another, the liver may fail to perform its vital functions. In the end, the organ as a whole comes under threat, begins to shrink, and then stops working altogether.

If you have cirrhosis caused by hepatitis C, your liver can degenerate as if you were drinking a bottle of whisky a day. It may well be that you are abstaining completely from all alcohol and drugs, and yet your liver is dissipating at an alarming rate. As the scarring progresses, there are fewer and fewer normal cells left, and these are put under more and more strain from the virus. The disease chips away at the healthy remains of your liver like a parasite draining its host of life-blood.

If the virus remains unchecked, then a cirrhotic liver is thought to be likely to fail within two to ten years. This estimate is based upon the figure for the mortality rate of people with all forms of active cirrhosis. According to this figure, 50 per cent of patients will be dead within five years of the onset of cirrhosis if the cause of the scarring is not halted or slowed.

The good news is that if treatment eliminates or retards the virus, then a cirrhotic liver can survive indefinitely. The liver is remarkably resilient, and only fails after a very large

14

proportion of its tissue is destroyed. Many people can live happily despite large amounts of scarring in the liver.

Hepatitis and Quality of Life

The overall effect of having some or all of the symptoms of hepatitis C is that your horizons shrink as inexorably as a cirrhotic liver. The switch from a happy, healthy, unbounded existence to a significantly reduced quality and expectation of life may leave you frightened and angry. This is both a point of despair and a point of departure. Some people will give in and give up. Some will just ignore the problem and hope that it goes away. Others will seek help and attempt to live with their problem in a constructive manner. Our intention is to show how this can be done.

Conclusion

There are two levels to the hepatitis C problem: one is personal, the other global. For anyone who is chronically infected, the disease can lead to serious liver damage and possibly death. For the community as a whole, hepatitis C is a viral legacy, which is slowly destroying the health of large numbers of the world population.

If you have the infection, it is worth recalling Francis Bacon's maxim that knowledge is power. The more you know, the better informed your strategies can be. By learning all you can about your disease, you will give yourself a useful start in coping successfully with hepatitis C.

2

How is Hepatitis C Diagnosed?

The process of detecting and evaluating a case of hepatitis C can take several months to complete and includes a number of blood tests, a liver biopsy, and consideration of your past medical history. At the end of the diagnosis, an impression forms of the nature and consequences of your condition. A liver specialist, or 'hepatologist', can then alert you to the possible dangers and can recommend treatment, if it is required.

Undergoing diagnosis can be psychologically draining. As more and more tests are done, and a stream of technical jargon is fired at you, a sense of confusion and bewilderment is likely to take over. The way to become clear-headed again is to find out precisely what it is that you have got, and how badly you have got it.

Why be Tested?

People are tested for HCV for many reasons. The majority are tested because they feel ill for no apparent reason, or because they fall into a risk category. Some are tested as part of a routine medical examination or as part of the screening procedure that blood donors undergo. In the

United Kingdom, a government-sponsored 'look back' exercise is currently underway to identify people with HCV, who donated blood before routine testing was introduced. The recipients of blood given by donors, who were unknowingly infected with HCV, are being identified and contacted so that testing for HCV can be undertaken.

A very few people find themselves being diagnosed in the strangest of circumstances. Christoff, 41, an antiques dealer from Dorset, felt dreadful without knowing what was wrong:

> 'About four years ago, I started feeling very ill. My main symptom was fatigue – everything was an effort. Even shaving tired me out. I also had very bad headaches and I had shivering . . . I felt cold and nauseous.
>
> 'It just so happened that my wife and I were trying to have a baby and she had gone to see a faith healer. The faith healer always sees the husband once. This woman did her thing of running her hands over my body. When she'd finished she said I'd got serious liver disease and I should do something about it.
>
> 'I went to my doctor and asked him to perform some liver tests. When the results came back, he told me I'd got aggressive hepatitis C.'

You do not need the ministrations of a faith healer to receive a reliable diagnosis. What you must do is consider whether you fall into any of the following categories. If you do, then you should consider being tested.

Blood Recipients

Anyone who received blood products before 1991 should consider being checked for HCV, since it is a blood-borne disease. It is believed that only a small number of HCV patients donated blood and that the number of infected units of blood inadvertently transfused into patients is therefore extremely small.

The risk of catching HCV from a transfusion is quite low for those who have received small quantities of blood, but rises sharply for patients who have been given large amounts. Accident victims and those who have had serious operations or have been in intensive care are at particular risk.

Former or Current Drug Users

If you have ever taken drugs by means of an injection, then you may have been infected by HCV. Regular intravenous users who share hypodermics or other equipment, run a high risk of infection. Even those who injected drugs just once or twice as an experiment, perhaps many years ago, are vulnerable. It is estimated that up to 70 per cent of current or former drug users are infected with HCV.

Inhaled Drugs

If you have ever inhaled ('snorted' or 'sniffed') drugs then you may still be at risk from hepatitis C. It has been shown that snorting drugs, for example, cocaine, heroin or speed, can transmit the virus through infected blood stuck to the end of a rolled-up note. However, this route of transmission is not very common.

Recipients of Certain Kinds of Medical Treatment Abroad

If you were taken ill in a third world country and given any blood tests or serum products, then you are at risk. You may also risk infection by having injections or acupuncture in some countries, since not all overseas medical services have adequate sterilization practices.

Haemophiliacs

Members of this group whose blood lacks an essential clotting agent and who are dependent on treatment with a concentrated clotting factor derived from donated blood, are routinely checked for viral infections.

Friends, Relations, Lovers, Colleagues and Carers of Any of the Above
The chances of infection at second hand are slight, but not unknown. If you do not fall into any of the above categories but have come into contact with someone with hepatitis C, then there is a risk of infection. Transmission may occur through tattooing, body-piercing, sharing razors or tooth-brushes, or unprotected penetrative sex – though it is some comfort to know that in northern Europe and North America most sexual partners of people with hepatitis C test negative for the antibody (see Chapter 4). Health care workers are vulnerable to accidents with needles.

The Tests Essential for a Diagnosis

To determine whether you have chronic hepatitis C you will need to undergo some or all of a variety of tests.

The Antibody Test
This is normally the first test that is performed. It involves taking a blood sample which is then examined for HCV antibodies. Antibodies are proteins that are made by the body to help fight infection. There are specific antibodies for each particular infection, so the presence of antibodies against HCV indicates that you have been exposed to the virus.

The antibody test is relatively cheap and is technically easy to perform. It is used as a screening test to separate those people who are definitely not infected from those who require more investigation. The antibody test measures only *exposure to* hepatitis C; many people who have been exposed to hepatitis C are not actually infected and will not develop any serious liver problems.

If your antibody test result is negative, you are free of the antibodies and no more tests are required. If your test result is positive, further investigation is essential.

The Polymerase Chain Reaction Test (PCR)
In this test, a sample of blood is analyzed for the presence of the virus. This is technically a very difficult procedure, as the virus is present in only minute amounts in the bloodstream, and in order to identify it the tiny amounts of virus that are present have to be amplified several million times. As a consequence, it is both an expensive test and not very reliable. Wrong results are not uncommon and the PCR test should always be interpreted with caution. Most hepatologists like to perform at least two PCR tests before they are confident about the result.

If your result is negative, then you appear to have cleared the virus, although the antibodies will remain in your bloodstream. This does not imply that you are immune to hepatitis C, since you can be re-infected.

Although the PCR test for hepatitis C is very sensitive it is sometimes not sensitive enough. A few people have very small amounts of virus in the blood which can rise and fall over time. It is therefore possible to be infected with hepatitis C and have such small amounts of virus that the PCR test shows that you are not infected. Normally the levels of virus in the blood change with time so that a second PCR test may reveal the true position. For this reason most doctors like to repeat a negative PCR test at least once just to be sure that this is a true negative. If you are tested negative by PCR for hepatitis C, you should not assume that you do not have the virus until the confirmatory tests have been performed.

A positive test result signifies that you are chronically infected with HCV. You are said to be 'HCV positive'.

Liver Function Tests (LFTs)

Anyone who has chronic hepatitis C needs an assessment of the general condition of his or her liver. This is usually obtained by performing liver function tests (LFTs), which are a series of tests performed on a single sample of blood. Usually, four or five measurements are made on the same sample. Each test provides slightly different information.

The two LFTs most commonly referred to are the alanine aminotransferase activity (ALT) and the aspartate aminotransferase activity (AST), which are jointly referred to as 'transaminases'. These measure the amounts of certain enzymes in the blood. Normally these enzymes are only found in liver cells, but if a liver cell is damaged, for example by a viral infection, the enzymes leak out and make their way into the blood where they can be detected. Thus the levels of ALT and AST in the blood indicate the amount of inflammation of the liver. However, in chronic HCV infection the amount of inflammation in the liver can change over time. The ALT and AST levels may be very high for some months and then return to normal. A few weeks later they may rise again. As a result of these fluctuations, measuring the blood ALT and AST is not a very good way of assessing how much liver damage has occurred. The main purpose of these tests is to provide a snapshot of what is going on in the liver at a single moment. Repeat testing of ALT and AST gives an indication of what is happening in the liver. If levels are persistently normal then it is likely that there is relatively little inflammation, but if they are always very high then it is most probable that the hepatitis is severe.

The LFTs also test blood products that indicate how well the liver is performing its vital functions. These tests measure how well the liver is clearing toxins from the blood (by measuring the serum bilirubin) and how much protein the liver is making (by measuring the serum albumin concentration). Both of these tests produce abnormal results in advanced liver disease (cirrhosis), although results can be normal even when the liver is badly scarred, because the liver has an enormous reserve capacity.

In addition to the standard LFTs, doctors sometimes measure the prothrombin index (PTI), which indicates how many clotting proteins the liver is making. This test complements the measurement of serum albumin.

Liver Biopsy
A worrying feature of liver disease is that the organ may function quite well and yet be badly damaged – just as a car engine may perform efficiently when you press the accelerator and still be rusty and about to seize up. In the car, only a thorough inspection under the bonnet will give the full picture. Similarly, in order to identify any structural abnormalities in the liver, a sample of tissue needs to be obtained and scrutinised under a microscope. This enables a specialist to assess the degree of any damage.

A biopsy involves taking a sliver of tissue directly from the liver by means of a special needle. It is pushed through the skin on the upper right side of the abdomen. The test is carried out while you are lying down, and you will be given a local anaesthetic to numb the area into which the needle is inserted. You may be offered valium to keep you calm during the procedure.

After the biopsy is over you will need to rest for several hours and have your blood pressure taken regularly during this period. There is a small possibility of damage to the liver causing internal bleeding (approximately one case in every 1,000 suffers a serious complication) which may require an operation to repair.

You will be warned by the doctor that the area surrounding the point of penetration of the needle tends to hurt when the anaesthetic wears off. In addition, you may feel an ache in the right shoulder. This is known as 'referred pain'. Nevertheless, most people feel only minor discomfort during and after a liver biopsy. Some do have bad experiences, most often when repeated penetration of the liver is necessary to obtain the correct amount of tissue.

You should think very carefully about what you are doing before having a biopsy. It is an invasive procedure, that is, one that involves medical intrusion into the body, with the risk, albeit small, of complications. Obtain information from your specialist and talk to people who have undergone the procedure (try to talk to several, so that you do not get just one view). Then discuss the issue with someone you trust. This should put you into a position in which you can make a fully informed decision.

Additional Tests

Ultrasound Scan of the Liver
A scan is a type of X-ray test, similar to that carried out on pregnant women to show the foetus inside the womb. Sound waves are bounced off the internal organs, enabling an image to be built up. For hepatitis patients, a scan helps to identify scarring or any other abnormalities in the liver, including cancerous tumours. The ultrasound test can detect gross abnormalities in the liver, but cannot determine the degree of inflammation that has occurred; nor can it identify minor degrees of scarring.

If a suspicious area is detected on ultrasound further X-rays will be taken, including whole body (CT or MRI) scans. This involves the patient lying in a tube while special images of the liver are produced.

Ultrasound is sometimes used to assist in performing a liver biopsy if there is difficulty finding the correct place to insert the needle. In this situation the ultrasonographer creates an image of the liver using ultrasound and guides the biopsy accordingly. Occasionally, this sort of biopsy is performed to ensure that a particular area of liver is sampled, for example when there is suspicion that a certain area of the liver may contain a small cancer.

Genotyping of the Virus
This is a procedure that is performed only by certain specialized research units. It consists of determining which of many subcategories ('genotypes') of HCV a particular strain falls into (see p.6 above). In the past determining the genotype was principally a research procedure, but it has become a determining factor in the duration of treatment by interferon and ribavirin (see Chapter 7).

Quantitative Viraemia Tests
This is another test that only a few hospitals carry out. Its purpose is to measure the amount of HCV within the bloodstream. Some experts use this information to assess the likely response to treatment, although there is controversy about how reliable this technique is. Once treatment has been completed, the test can indicate its success or failure.

The Emotional Response to a Positive Diagnosis

Discovering that you have chronic hepatitis tends to provoke a mixture of relief and shock. You may feel relief because you finally have an explanation of why you have felt ill for such a long time. Perhaps you have been misdiagnosed in the past, or doctors have been unable to attribute your condition to any particular cause. At the same time, you may be horrified at having hepatitis C. Finding out that you have a virus that threatens a vital organ and could be fatal often leads to blind panic. It is natural to fear death, and a positive diagnosis taps this deep-rooted insecurity.

Feyona, a Scottish housewife, was painfully relieved to find out that she had hepatitis C after years of misdiagnosis:

'Five years ago I thought I may as well give up. I had joint pains and chronic tiredness and had been diagnosed as having RA (rheumatoid arthritis), a death sentence to someone as fit and active as me. Three years before that it was thought I might have ME (myalgic encephalitis), and somewhere in between I had hurt my back. I was giving up hope of finding out what was wrong. I knew I just didn't feel right.

'I moved house and the new hospital I attended had a liver specialist with an interest in rheumatology. He wasn't convinced I had RA. I remember him telling me several tests later that he would check me for hepatitis C. I waited six weeks and found that I was positive.'

Christoff was pleased that he did not have anything more serious when he discovered he had hepatitis C. This gave way to shock once he realized that he had a long-term illness:

'My initial reaction was relief because I thought I'd got something terminal. I thought it was leukaemia or something like that. So when the doctor told me it was hepatitis C and explained what it was, although I took upon board the seriousness of my situation, I felt a certain amount of relief.

'Then the consequences of having a chronic infection slowly got through to me. I was in a state of shock for quite a while after finding out.'

Katherine, a mother of two from London, was frightened by her positive diagnosis:

'Knowing that I had chronic hepatitis absolutely terrified me. I have always been very worried about my health. Because I used to be a nurse I understood a little bit about what this meant and a little bit of knowledge was probably not good for me. I also didn't really know anyone else at that time who had it.'

Post-Diagnosis Counselling

On being diagnosed as having chronic hepatitis C, you will need counselling. This is usually offered by the doctor who informs you of your condition. The initial counselling session will cover the following points:

- The significance of having chronic hepatitis C.
- How long you may have had the virus. A blood transfusion in the past or a history of intravenous drug use will be relevant in making an estimate.
- An outline of the course and dangers of the disease. Those with a mild form of the disease are told that they may never develop serious liver problems, although they will require lifelong observation to ensure that the liver remains well. Those with aggressive liver disease are warned about the dangers relating to their particular condition. Someone with cirrhosis has a worse prognosis than someone without.

- Agreement on an appropriate plan of action. This will map out what further investigation, monitoring and check-ups are advisable, and summarize the kinds of treatment available.
- Referral to a specialist unit if you are not already attending one. Departments dealing with hepatitis C are generally located at teaching hospitals.
- Introduction to a local support group. The London teaching hospitals, the British Liver Trust, the Haemophilia Society or Mainliners (an organisation that helps drug users) can tell you about your local group. (See the section on 'Useful Addresses' at the end of this book for details.)
- How to obtain information about HCV, for example, from pamphlets on hepatitis issued by the drug companies or the British Liver Trust.
- Consideration of any lifestyle factors which may be suggested by your diagnosis. For instance, if you are a heavy drinker it is a good idea to cut down on your alcohol intake.

It is worth planning for your initial counselling session to avoid becoming confused or not getting the most out of it. Two strategies in particular are useful. First, you may find it helpful to take a friend or relation with you to see the doctor. A companion gives moral support and can check your understanding of the diagnosis and recommendations. Second, it is a good idea to prepare questions that you would like answered in advance of the appointment. Write them down and go through them with someone you trust. This way you can make sure that you receive clear information that is pertinent to your case.

Living with the Uncertainty
of Having Chronic Hepatitis C

Having received your diagnosis and attended your initial counselling session, you may be overwhelmed by the precariousness of your situation. Although you can be sure that you now have a dangerous virus, you cannot be certain of the consequences for you or your friends and family. You do not know if you are going to get better. You do not know if you are going to get cirrhosis or cancer. You cannot predict how other people you care about will be affected. All you can be sure of is that you have a serious illness.

Finding out that you have chronic hepatitis C changes your life. Part of that change consists in going through a series of emotional reactions.

Shock and Denial

Taking on board the idea that you have a chronic disease involves a grieving process. Your initial reaction is likely to be a mixture of numbing astonishment and disbelief. You may become frozen and unable to comprehend what has been said to you at your various appointments. If so, take it slowly. You may only be able to absorb a little information at a time.

On thinking about your new status, you may well recoil with disbelief. William, a 39-year-old company director, attempted to deny and minimize his problem:

'I thought there had been a terrible mistake. How could I have hepatitis C? I wanted all the tests checked and double-checked to make sure.

'Then I denied the seriousness of my complaint. I said to myself: "It's trivial. Thousands of people have got hepatitis and come to no harm."

'The trouble was, my biopsy indicated extensive liver damage and I needed to make some changes in my lifestyle in order to preserve it.

'Very gradually, I have awakened to the reality of having a long-term illness which undermines the quality of my life.'

Fear and Sadness

When the truth begins to dawn on you, fear is likely to emerge. Having a serious disease creates anxiety: 'Am I going to die? Will I get cancer? Will my liver fail?'

The therapy for fear is faith. The worst thing to do is to crumple up and hide away. Tell your friends about your worries. Find other people with hepatitis C and discuss your concerns with them. They will probably identify with you in a sympathetic way and help to lighten your load.

You will also go through phases of sadness. You have lost your health and need to mourn its passing away. Just as you may cry at the funeral of a relative or friend, so you need to allow yourself to express your personal anguish about being ill.

Anger, Blame and Defiance

Believing that you have chronic hepatitis C almost always causes boiling rage: 'I'm furious I've got this virus!'

You will probably try to blame non-specific as well as identified targets for your misfortune: 'I want to kill whoever gave me this infection! I bet it was that doctor on holiday last year who contaminated me.'

Anger and blame are parts of the defiance stage of the cycle of reactions. These emotional responses are understandable: no one wants to be chronically ill. A way to deal with them is to allow yourself to be upset and to recognize that it is part of a healthy response to a tough situation.

Unwelcome – and Welcome – Isolation
A problem for many who have a serious illness is the tendency to isolation. It is dangerous to drop too far into the slough of despond. If you become severely depressed, it is a good idea to talk things over with your doctor or specialist. Some form of medication, such as antidepressants, may be appropriate.

However, there may be times when you simply want to be left alone to reflect on your situation. You may temporarily withdraw from your usual routine. This can be a period of healthy self-appraisal, but partners, friends and family may find it hard to cope with. It will be easier for them if you tell them that although you do not want to talk about your illness at the moment, you will when you are ready.

Conclusion

Going through the various stages of diagnosis is an emotional assault course. Having the tests and waiting for the results raise all kinds of anxieties. Discovering that you have chronic hepatitis C is a profound shock.

When you work through the feelings attached to your new status, you will eventually experience peace of mind. This marks the transition from denial and anger to acceptance. Understanding the reality of HCV and how serious your particular case is will help to lessen the fear sparked off by your diagnosis. A proper sense of proportion will re-emerge and you will be strong enough to face the consequences of your illness.

3

How to Stop the
Hepatitis C Virus Spreading

Having been diagnosed with hepatitis C, you are responsible for making sure that you do not infect anyone else. The way to protect the world at large is to take certain precautions in your day-to-day life. Initially, these may feel restrictive, but to know that you are doing your best to prevent a dangerous disease from spreading has its own rewards.

People have to trust you not to infect them. They are at your mercy, since they cannot know that you carry the virus unless you tell them and, in many circumstances, it is not appropriate to announce the fact. In a sense you are powerful, especially in situations where other people are unaware of your infection. You can choose not to put others at risk by following some simple guidelines, or you can be sloppy about the precautions, and so possibly cause harm.

Recognizing that you are infectious may make you feel differently about yourself in some ways. Often, patients feel dirty and lose confidence in social and sexual relationships. Sometimes families, friends and colleagues inadvertently reinforce this perception. Others experience only support and love from those close to them. It is important for you to reconstruct your self-esteem, and acting responsibly to avoid spreading infection can help you in this process.

Basic Dos and Don'ts

There are certain definite steps you can take to prevent the spread of hepatitis C. Remember, you have a dangerous, active virus in your bloodstream. Unless you are vigilant, others may catch it from you.

- Do not share razors, toothbrushes or other intimate items.
- Clean up any blood spills immediately with household bleach, which kills the hepatitis C virus very efficiently.
- Be careful with bloodstained tissues, tampons and so on. Make sure you dispose of them properly by placing them in a plastic bag in the dustbin.
- Cover cuts and wounds with waterproof dressings as soon as possible.
- Tell your partner you have HCV and explain the dangers of having hepatitis. Your partner may want to be tested if you have had unprotected sex together, as there is the possibility of transmission during sexual contact, although it is extremely small.
- Wear condoms during penetrative sex. There are male and female varieties (see below).
- Avoid sexual contact during and immediately after your period if you are a female patient. HCV has been found in menstrual blood.
- Tell your doctor (if he or she does not already know), dentist and any other health care worker you see that

you have hepatitis C. Anyone who may be exposed to your blood is at risk.

- Do not donate blood or register as an organ donor.
- Do not share needles or equipment if you are a drug user.
- Do not get tattooed or body-pierced.

HCV and Sex

Sexual Transmission of the Virus
It is possible for HCV to be transmitted sexually. It is a fact that the virus is more widespread among people who are sexually promiscuous than among those who are not. The medical profession concludes that there is a risk of infection by this means.

However, it is a relatively rare and inefficient route of transmission. Scientists cannot prove that bodily fluids other than blood transmit HCV. The danger probably lies not in the exchange of sexual substances, but in the passage of blood within them. For example, if you have an internal cut and bleed into your sexual fluids, then there is a risk. Studies of long-term relationships where one partner is infected with HCV show that the frequency of transmission to the other partner is low; but it is *not* nil.

Different hospitals take different views about the risk. In London, St Mary's, Paddington, argues for safe sex even within stable partnerships – except in the event of a couple wanting to have a baby. On the other hand, the Royal Free Hospital, Hampstead, considers that 'there is no logic for couples in long-standing relationships to begin barrier sexual practices after diagnosis.'

To be on the safe side, it is recommended that anyone who is sexually active should use condoms for all sexual contact, except for purposes of conception. This keeps the chance of infection to an absolute minimum.

Attitudes towards Sex
Having a sexually transmissible disease alters your attitude towards making love. You may think that no one will ever want to sleep with you again for fear of catching the virus. You may also think that using condoms will destroy the pleasure of the intimate act.

William became insecure about finding a sexual partner after being diagnosed with hepatitis C. As he illustrates, the way to combat anxiety about safe sex is to be open and honest with your partner:

'When the sister at the hospital said that the virus might be sexually transmissible and that I should employ safe sex, I worried that I would never sleep with anyone ever again.

'On holiday I met Celine, a French woman with whom I fell in love. She was attracted to me and I hoped things would go further. When it became clear that we wanted to sleep with each other I told her that I had hepatitis C. Her immediate reaction was blind fear. She valued her health and did not want to jeopardize it as she had children to look after. I was crestfallen as I thought she had rejected me.

'After we discussed the use of condoms and the fact that hepatitis C only passes in blood, not in semen or other bodily fluids, our anxieties subsided. Some time later nature ran her course and we made love employing safe sex. I was delighted to be accepted in spite of my disease.'

Using Condoms
Before being advised to practise safe sex, you may never have thought about using condoms. They are safe because

they offer barrier protection against sexually transmitted diseases as well as providing effective contraception. Condoms are suitable for most couples. There are male and female varieties. A male condom is a narrow tube made from very thin latex rubber, with a teat at the closed end to catch the semen once the man has ejaculated. It is soft and stretchy, and looks and behaves a bit like a child's balloon.

A female condom is a sheath made of very thin rubber or polyurethane plastic. It is closed at one end and is designed to form a loose lining to a woman's vagina. There are two flexible rings, one at each end of the condom, to keep it in place. The ring at the closed end fits inside the vagina behind the pubic bone. The ring at the open end stays outside, placed against the area around the vulva.

In making a decision about whether to use the male or female variety, one suggestion is that the partner with the infection takes the precaution. After all, the moral onus is on the patient not to spread the virus. Another thought is that the partner who does not have the virus might prefer to be in control and so feel happier being the one who wears the condom.

A common fear is that condoms inhibit the spontaneity and sensuality of lovemaking. What could be more disconcerting than trying to fit a prophylactic device over your genitals in the midst of your passion? Another worry is that condoms will reduce the pleasure derived from penetrative sex, interposing a layer of rubber between you and the complete nakedness of your partner. However, as you practise safe sex, you will find that it is something that can easily be incorporated into your love life. Putting on condoms can even be fun, and hardly anyone finds that they detract from sexual arousal. With a little love, safe sex can become a mutually caring process like the intimate act itself.

How to use a male condom   You can obtain male condoms from your doctor, family planning clinic or chemist. You may be told how to use them, or you can ask. Instructions are generally given on the outside of the pack or in a leaflet inside it. Key points to remember are:

- Use a condom every time you engage in penetrative sex.
- Never use a condom more than once.
- Put the condom on before there is any contact between the penis and the vaginal area, because fluid released during the early stages of arousal can contain sperm.
- The penis must be erect before the condom is put on. The man can put on the condom himself, or his partner can do it.
- Be careful not to tear the condom with sharp fingernails or jewellery.
- During penetration, you must ensure that the condom stays on. If it begins to come off, then put it back on again properly. If it comes off completely, then start again with a fresh condom.
- After orgasm, withdraw the penis from the vagina and remove the condom before the penis has gone completely soft.
- Wrap the condom in some tissue and dispose of it. It is best not to use the lavatory as a condom does not always flush away properly.

How to use a female condom   To obtain female condoms, you should go to a family planning clinic, where the nurse or doctor will explain how to use them. The pack also contains a set of instructions. Key points to remember are:

- Use a new condom each time you make love.
- Insert the condom any time before penetrative sex. It must be in place before the man's penis touches the

woman's genital area as fluid, which may contain sperm, can seep out before ejaculation.

- Put the condom in when you are lying down, squatting, or with one leg on a stool or chair. Try out different ways until you find the most comfortable one for you. The condom can be inserted by either partner.
- Take the condom out of the pack carefully, being sure not to damage it with jewellery or fingernails.
- Be certain that the outer ring rests closely against the vulva.
- When preparing for penetration, it is suggested that the woman guide the man's penis into the condom to ensure that it does not slip around it and so directly into the vagina.
- After intercourse, take out the condom, twisting the outer ring to keep the semen inside.
- Dispose of the condom by wrapping it in tissue and placing it in a bin.

Hepatitis and Parenthood

If you or your partner have hepatitis C and you want to have a baby, you need to be able to make an informed decision about how to proceed. This involves understanding the risks and dangers of passing on the infection to your offspring.

What is the Risk of Transmission?
The effects of HCV in children are not yet fully understood. Some authorities hold that infected children have aggressive disease, while others believe that the infection can also be mild in young children. Perhaps it is comforting to know that doctors do not yet understand what HCV does to children because very few children with HCV have

been identified. This clearly indicates that transmission of HCV from parents to their offspring is uncommon.

Father-to-child transmission at conception is unheard-of. The danger lies in mother-to-child infection, which does occur but rarely. Transmission is more likely to take place where the mother has a high concentration of HCV in her bloodstream. This is rare in most patients with a single viral infection, but common in mothers who are also HIV positive.

The way in which HCV can be transmitted to children is still being studied. Some hepatologists speculate that the HCV virus may be able to cross the placenta and enter the baby's body while the infant is still in the womb. Another theory is that the virus may be transmitted to the baby during childbirth, for example, when the mother's blood comes into contact with the baby.

If the infection can only be transmitted during childbirth, then it may be appropriate to deliver all mothers with HCV by Caesarian section. If the virus is transmitted during the baby's time in the womb, then clearly this is not the answer. At present the risk of transmission of HCV from mothers to their babies is so low that most experts agree it is unnecessary to perform Caesarian sections on all women with HCV.

A similar situation applies to breast-feeding. Specialists do not know whether this practice can pass the virus on to infants. Since the vast majority of babies who are fed in this way by their infected mothers do not catch HCV, the risk, if any, must be small. Most experts agree that mothers with HCV should be encouraged to breast-feed because of the enormous advantages for both mother and infant.

Christoff, whose wife has hepatitis C, expresses justified concern about passing on the disease to his offspring:

'Both my wife and I have hepatitis C. When we were considering having a baby, the possibility of transmitting the virus to our child was a major concern. The hospital told us that about one in a hundred positive women have babies that are infected . . . It was the most appalling thought that we could bring this little mite into the world and sentence it to a life with hepatitis C.'

Once your baby has been born, you and your partner may wish to consider testing to check that your infant has not contracted HCV. As it can take some time for the virus to become detectable in the child, testing should be delayed for a few weeks or months after birth. Most doctors test for HCV when the baby is three to six months old. In the vast majority of cases your baby will be found to be HCV negative. If your baby is found to be infected, then it is important to get early medical advice from a doctor who has experience in treating children with HCV.

Avoiding Infection after Birth
You must remember that you are still carrying the virus and that transmission to your child is possible. Passing it on during normal kissing and cuddling is unheard-of, but your blood is potentially infectious. The simple dos and don'ts listed above are very important when young children are in the house. It is worth recalling that children's fingers go everywhere, so take special care to clean up carefully if you spill any of your blood and be careful to cover any cuts or scratches with a sticking-plaster.

Taking a Balanced View
If you or your partner carries the virus, the sensible approach is to think very carefully about having a child and to discuss it with your doctor. Although the risk of parent–child infection is small, it is not entirely negligible.

The possibility of this route of transmission and the consequences for a baby with hepatitis C must be taken into account. Your decision should be based on an informed judgement.

Should you be extremely unlucky and your baby be infected, it is natural to feel guilty. You should remember that your child was a wanted child, conceived with love and care, and that you and your partner did everything possible to stop your child becoming infected.

HCV Infection and your Relationships

How you perceive yourself and how others perceive you can alter radically as a result of having a chronic infection. This in turn can lead to a transformation of your attitude to others and their responses to you.

Close relationships are particularly vulnerable when you have a long-term illness. At first, your self-image gets a terrible hammering and you think that no one wants, needs or loves you any more.

The best way to cope with a sudden fall in self-esteem is to discuss your insecurities with your partner and family. Single people who lack a system of support can turn deeper and deeper into themselves, thinking that they will be an unwelcome burden to any potential partner or friend. Katherine became convinced that no one wanted her because of her hepatitis:

'Just to know that I've got a dangerous virus makes me feel unclean. It also makes me feel less desirable and less good a prospect for any sort of man that might come my way. I think, not only am I a single mother with two children and on the wrong side of forty, but I also have a chronic illness.'

The way to combat the lowering of perceived attrac-
tiveness is to recognize your intrinsic worth. This trans-
cends the idea of being 'damaged' or 'soiled goods'. Your
having an illness is an external factor, and need not
influence your capacity for loving or being loved. After
all, Katherine's children love her regardless of her hepatitis.

The Danger of a 'Leper Mentality'
Some people, when diagnosed with hepatitis C, turn into
themselves and adopt what can be called a 'leper mentality'. You feel alone with your problem and that no one
cares about you. You expect rejection because of your
disease and become more and more isolated.

Sometimes there is an element of reality in this fear.
Friends and relatives may become anxious and resentful
when you tell them that you have a serious virus. They hate
the fact that you are ill and the changes your infection
makes to their lives. Partners will naturally enough be
concerned about the possibility of sexual transmission.
Spouses will be concerned about the danger of passing
on the virus to any children you have planned or already
have.

Some people may be unsympathetic and stigmatize you,
encouraging the idea that you are unclean because of your
chronic disease. Your having a virus evokes a fear which
feeds on ignorance and prejudice.

Chris, 59, a playwright from Hampstead, was ostracized
when he was open about his illness:

'I told some old friends I'd got hep C and at one point
they asked me not to visit them. They happened to be
blood donors and the place where they gave blood
forbade them to mix socially with HCV infectious
people. Such contact might cast doubt on the purity
of their donation.

'I felt like a marked man. I felt I'd been made into a pariah. And then I got very angry . . . because it was a real rejection.'

You may be treated with suspicion in other ways that you find hurtful. You may notice people being wary about their cups, glasses and cutlery after you use them. You may find parents not allowing their children to play with yours.

A useful strategy in dealing with prejudice is to let your friends and loved ones get on with their adjustment to your illness. This takes time, and everyone has their own method of doing it. On occasion, you may need to challenge someone's treatment of you if it goes too far. Perseverance, and educating others about hepatitis, are the best ways of dispelling ignorance and bias.

Tracy, from Southampton, is the mother of Cathryn, 9, who was infected with hepatitis C when she received immunoglobulin therapy for her auto-immune disorder. At school Cathryn was misunderstood and rejected because of her infection:

'I (Tracy) told the school that Cathryn had hepatitis C and they didn't have a clue what I was on about. One day Cathryn was ill, and she was left in the corridor for half an hour until I came to pick her up.

'The teachers were funny about cuts. If Cathryn bled . . . even a graze on the knee . . . they wouldn't touch her. They called me and put her in isolation until I got there.

'The other children teased Cathryn, saying she'd got AIDS or blood poisoning. When they all went to the beach, the mothers wouldn't let Cathryn drink from the same cups or use the same knives and forks.

'Since all this happened, I have moved Cathryn to a

new school, where she receives proper medical assistance and understanding from the staff.'

Conclusion

You have a duty not to spread hepatitis C. It is an infectious disease that can be passed to your offspring as well as among your peer group. Protecting others requires you to take various common-sense precautions, none of which radically compromises your lifestyle.

You may meet with fear and prejudice in others. They may view you as somehow unclean for being infectious. Most will get over this attitude in time.

As you learn to take care not to spread the virus, your self-esteem will rise in the knowledge that you are taking responsibility for your disease. People will respect you for your desire to protect the people around you. Your regard for others says much about your humanity.

4

Day-to-Day Coping

If you experience no ill effects from your hepatitis C infection, you will probably want to skip this chapter. However, as we saw in Chapter 1, many of you with the virus experience tiredness, nausea and malaise. The end result is a drain on your energy. Work, social and family life, and sexuality can all suffer because you feel too listless to participate in and enjoy them to the full.

If one or more of these symptoms afflicts you, you can combat the erosion of your life by following some common-sense suggestions. The way to flourish in spite of the infection is to manage your lifestyle in an effective way. This involves finding the right balance between activity and rest, eating healthily, and building up a system of support.

Assessing the Impact of Hepatitis on Your Life

The first step on the road to coping successfully with hepatitis C is to understand the effects it has upon you. When you have become acquainted with your disease, you will be better able to cope with it. A clearly marked hurdle is far easier to jump than one which you cannot see clearly.

You can start to assess the limitations imposed on you by

hepatitis C by answering the following questions. Be honest: the answers are for you, not for anyone else.

Tiredness
- Do you feel tired a lot of the time?
- Is it very difficult for you to get up in the morning?
- Do you tend to feel tired when you used not to, whether at work or with your family?
- Are you too exhausted by the end of the day to go out in the evenings?
- Do you sleep for days on end?
- Do you take a nap at lunch time?
- Do you regularly sleep all day at the weekend or on your holidays?

Nausea
- Do you frequently feel sick?
- Do certain types of food make you nauseous?
- Do you ever regret eating fish and chips for supper? Or fried eggs and bacon for breakfast? Or curries?
- Does drinking small quantities of alcohol cause you unjustified hangovers?

Malaise
- Are you prone to catching whatever cold or flu is going around?
- Do you keep getting slight sore throats that go on for ever?
- Do you sweat a lot?
- Do you often feel depressed?
- Do you think that things can only get worse?
- Are your thoughts about people, places and things that you love painted in dark hues?
- Are you irritable?
- Do you snap at people without really knowing why?

Effects on Quality of Life
- Do you prefer to lie in front of the television rather than go out?
- Are the only appointments you make the ones you cannot avoid?
- Has your motivation declined?
- If you work, are you performing less diligently than before?
- If you are out of work, can you face trying to find a job?
- Do you derive less and less pleasure from your sexuality?
- Are you making love on fewer occasions than you used to?
- If you do not have a partner, can you be bothered to find one?
- Have you stopped masturbating?
- Are you worried that your interest in sex is declining?

If you answered 'Yes!' to some of the above questions, then you need to reconsider your lifestyle. Many chronic hepatitis patients answer positively to several in each section.

What you are doing here is pinpointing the ways in which active hepatitis is undermining your ability to enjoy a full life. By doing so, you are beginning to define the nature of the problem which confronts you; and understanding a problem is halfway to solving it.

Managing Your Lifestyle

Katherine describes how she copes with her fatigue:

'I get good days and bad days. I have to pace myself and do certain things in order to make myself feel well.

'If I ever stay out too late or push myself to the limit, it takes me maybe a week instead of just a good night's

49

sleep to get over it. I have to get proper rest, which is helped by going to bed at regular hours.

'I don't drink alcohol any more and I get regular exercise. I swim nearly every day and that helps me a lot, even though I don't feel like doing it very much.

'I have to really pay attention to my body's needs and do everything I can to obtain the best sort of health for myself in order to have a reasonable quality of life.'

Christoff improved his diet and reduced his stress levels in order to cope. He felt better almost immediately:

'Having been diagnosed with hepatitis C, I changed my lifestyle dramatically to try to do something about it. The first thing I did was to see a nutritionist, who did various tests on me to find out what I was deficient in. In particular, I lacked zinc and magnesium.

'I changed my diet. I cut out almost all dairy products, red meat, and coffee which I'd drunk like a maniac. Luckily, I'd stopped smoking some years before. I started to lead a much healthier life.

'I also cut down my stress levels. At the time I was diagnosed, my business was going bust and I was under the most appalling pressure. I consciously tried to lead a life that was less stressful. If I feel stressed out, then I start to feel ill.

'It paid off. I began to notice improvements quite quickly. I stopped feeling nauseous. Although I was still very tired, I had slightly more energy. I just felt better. Instinctively I knew I was benefiting from these changes.'

Fatigue and Sleep
If you feel unremittingly tired it is important to get proper rest. The first task is to establish a regular pattern of sleep at night.

To sleep well you must adopt a routine for yourself, as you would for a young child. Have hot chocolate or camomile tea in the late evening to calm yourself down. Go to bed and get up at regular times. For example, go to bed at 11.00 p.m. and get up at 7.30 a.m. If you sleep well, this will be enough to set you up for the day.

If you sleep badly at night, then you may need to 'catnap' during the day. A useful tactic is to adopt the continental habit of having a siesta after lunch. Should you require more rest than this, then you must adapt your daily routine accordingly.

It is essential that you recognize how much sleep you need, and when. It takes time to evaluate this, and the answer you come up with will be personal to you. It might be that eight hours a night plus a one-hour nap in the afternoon is enough for one person, while ten hours per night and no nap suits another.

The worst thing you can do is to neglect this aspect of your regimen. Making yourself even more tired will diminish your powers to enjoy life. For instance, some unmanageable individuals drink coffee all evening and then go to bed at three in the morning. Even if they did not have hepatitis, they would feel dreadful.

Levels of Activity
The treatment for malaise is to find the sensible point between doing too little and doing too much. If not managed properly, malaise can lead to malingering. You must guard against the danger of ending up as a couch potato.

The dilemma is that if you feel depressed and so disinclined to do very much, then you do less and less and become more and more downcast as a result, thus creating a downward spiral into despair.

An alternative problem is being tempted to do too

much. The more you do, the more depressed you become because your stress levels are taking off vertically. You enter an upwards whirlwind of hyperactivity from which you cannot come down. You become increasingly frustrated and doom-laden. The more you do, the less it satisfies you because of the rise in anxiety and tiredness.

In both predicaments the remedy is to strike a balance between under- and over-activity. To establish what is the right amount for you to do, you have to take your own circumstances into account. Gauge what you need to do and what you want to do, and offset these demands against what you can do. For example, you need to go shopping to buy your food. You may not like doing it, and so do not want to do it; but you can do it, since you are physically able and you have the time. If it takes a lot out of you, allow yourself a rest after each shopping trip. Learn how long you can spend at the shops without getting worn out.

Combating Stress

It is essential to deal with stress, not simply to ignore it. There are no universal solutions; all that can be said is that you must find a way to relax. Some find meditation or yoga helpful, or going for a swim each morning. Taking the dog for a walk or engaging in a pleasurable hobby are other possibilities. No one but yourself can legislate precisely what is right for you.

Diet

Diet is intimately related to your well-being. Eat the wrong things and you may feel worse; eat the right things and your diet will be a defence against your disease.

Some believe that a poor diet is the cause of the skin blemishes, headaches and joint pains that many hepatitis patients complain about. Even healthy people who eat the wrong foods get spots!

There is also a positive reason for adopting a healthy diet. Good nutrition, ensuring you get enough calories, proteins and fat, can help a damaged liver to generate new cells.

In general, it is best to avoid too much fat and oil, for example, fried food and full-cream dairy produce. It is advisable to eat lots of vegetables and fruit, and to get your protein from white fish or lean meat.

Foods to avoid include:

- *greasy*, e.g. fish in batter, chips, fatty meat, bacon, sausages, fried bread;
- *spicy*, e.g. curries, Mexican food, most far eastern cuisines;
- *sugary*, e.g. Chinese meals cooked in monosodium glutamate; fruit pies or crumbles; sweets, cakes, biscuits and chocolate;
- *creamy*, e.g. full-fat milk, cheese, yoghurt and ice-cream; rich puddings, sauces or gravy.

Concentrate instead on eating:

- *'diet', low fat or no added sugar and salt products*: any packet or tin with one or more of these prefixes added to the label, e.g. baked beans, cottage cheese, yoghurt, etc.;
- *vegetables*: any are beneficial, but greens such as cabbage, spinach and broccoli, as well as carrots, are particularly liver-friendly;
- *fruit*: apples, pears, oranges, pineapples, grapefruit and so on are all desirable;
- *meat and fish*: it is not so much what you eat in this category, but rather how you cook it; most kinds are fine so long as they are grilled or baked in foil in the oven.

Seek detailed advice on diet from people who have eaten in a healthy way for some time. They will know delicious and appropriate recipes and make sensible suggestions about where to buy the right produce. After a while, you will become your own expert in this field; taking an informed interest in healthy eating can be a source of pleasure and satisfaction in itself.

Sexuality
Your sex drive may suffer as a consequence of your hepatitis. If your partner does not have the virus, he or she may want to make love more often than you do. If you find this is the case, frank discussion is necessary to establish reasonable boundaries. Don't force yourself to be sexy when you don't feel like it. The sex instinct has a life of its own. You need to understand your desires and allow them to surface in their own way at their own time. You can be sure they will, even if perhaps not with the frequency and intensity you would ideally like.

Support Groups

In building foundations for a programme of self-help, you need to establish a system of factual and emotional support. The main thing is to find other people who have gone through the kinds of problems that you are currently facing. You can benefit from their experience, strength and hope.

A fruitful way of contacting other hepatitis patients is to attend a local support group, or if you cannot get there, to get in touch with its organizer. Making contact with other hepatitis patients will give you a peer group of people who will identify – and sympathize – with you.

Katherine found going to her local meeting extremely informative:

'It was really good. There were about eight people sitting on chairs in a loose circle. The guy running it was hep C positive and there were people in different stages of having the illness: some with mild disease, some with aggressive. We swapped stories, telling each other the different things we did in order to try and get well and how we coped with it. We talked about interferon treatment and the pros and cons of interferon. We were handed a lot of really good information about hep C, which I found incredibly helpful.'

Attending a support group can give you not only factual help – information and ideas – but also the emotional support which is so badly needed by anyone dealing with feelings about having hepatitis and the depressing effect of active disease.

Christoff made contacts at his support group and then kept in touch. If he needs help, he can pick up the phone and ask for it:

'I think it's a very hard thing to live with hepatitis without support. The disease is a frightening and over-powering bogeyman, which can pounce at any moment. It's at its most powerful when I think I am the only one who has got it.

'Becoming part of an informal network of other sufferers was a big help. I now have many friends who are fellow sufferers. I'm lucky, if that's the right word, to know a lot of people with it. I met almost all of them through a self-help group I attended in London and since then I've phoned them regularly.

'If I feel depressed, I ring a friend who is sympathetic. He will identify with my problem because he has it too, and has been through the same thing. Hopefully, he isn't having such a bad day as I am and will share with me a little of his strength.'

An important consequence of receiving such help is that after a while you will be able to pass on your own store of experience and wisdom to people who are at an earlier stage than you in the struggle with hepatitis. New members of the group will seek your assistance. Sharing your insights gives you a continually renewed role in a loving and caring process of mutual self-help.

Starting a Support Group

Many hepatitis patients seeking a support group cannot find one in the area in which they live. If this is your difficulty, why not try to form a local group? This is a service not just to yourself but to any other people in the district who find themselves frustrated in the attempt to establish links with fellow sufferers.

Publicity   Your first step must be to let people know that you are creating a support group; so you must advertise your meeting. Put up posters in doctors' surgeries, on hospital notice boards, and so on. Inform the medical carers of local hepatitis patients of what you are doing and they will pass on to their charges news of the meeting. In general, they will be very cooperative.

Venue   Once you have decided to set up a local support group, you need to find somewhere to hold the meeting. It should be somewhere safe, comfortable, and preferably near to public transport. Liver clinics, community projects, health education centres and similar institutions are often willing to provide a meeting room, or at least point you in the right direction for finding one.

Time and day of meeting   You need to set a regular time for meetings that will suit as many people as possible. For example, you may think that the second Wednesday of each month at 7.30 p.m. is convenient; but there may be people with children who cannot easily manage this. Only by talking with other people who want to attend can you settle on an arrangement that is convenient for most people.

Coverage   The aims of the group are likely to include:

- the sharing of information and experience (factual support);
- the sharing of the emotions aroused by having hepatitis (emotional support);
- discussion of lifestyle management;
- consideration of different treatments of hepatitis.

Counselling

It is not uncommon for people with chronic hepatitis to need individual counselling. The feelings aroused by having a chronic disease may be too much to handle on your own. Talking to a professional therapist can help to deal with some of the difficult emotions, particularly the fear and anger associated with discovering your condition.

If you need a counsellor, you can contact your local health authority for guidance as to how to find a professional, qualified in helping those with serious illness handle their emotions. You should try to identify a counsellor with experience in dealing with patients who have HCV – though as the virus has only been identified fairly recently this may not be all that easy.

Ideally, you will meet your counsellor in a secure place

on a regular basis. He or she will listen to what you say and then give some appropriate feedback. You will grow in confidence, so that you are able to be completely open about your feelings. Through revealing them to someone experienced in dealing with such problems, you will learn to live with your disease at the emotional level.

Conclusion

Although you will have your own, unique physical and psychological responses to having hepatitis C, there are certain shared features on which guidance is available. If you are too fatigued or ache-ridden to live to your maximum potential, a strategy of vigilance over levels of activity, diet and emotional support can help to improve your quality of life.

The key is to assess how the disease affects you and then to follow the dictates of common-sense. You can reap noticeable rewards from managing your lifestyle. You can do the things that you choose to do with satisfaction and gusto. You no longer feel a slave to hepatitis; to some extent you become its master. Most of all, you can take pride in being responsible for your attitude to your condition.

5

Treatment with Prescribed Drugs

Many of you with hepatitis C are advised by a specialist to take a course of prescribed medication. The aim of treatment is to eliminate the virus, leaving you free of infection and its consequences.

Using the latest treatments, approximately 40 per cent of patients clear the virus completely, and many who are not cured receive a temporary benefit. Those who do not respond to initial therapy may be re-treated at a later date or advised to wait for further advances in the treatment of hepatitis C.

A course of medication provokes a spectrum of side-effects, which can be marked, although many patients find them tolerable. Difficult to handle is the psychological impact, for patients often become depressed. However, those who complete treatment and enjoy a long-term response feel more than compensated for suffering its short-term rigours.

Why a Doctor Recommends Treatment

In general, a hepatologist recommends treatment for anyone with moderate to severe liver disease due to HCV. In arriving at his or her decision, the specialist takes several medical factors into account. These relate to the severity of your liver disease and your expected ability to tolerate interferon alpha, which is the main ingredient in therapies for chronic HCV. This drug is associated with a number of side-effects and is expensive, costing several thousands pounds per annum.

Most specialists agree that because taking interferon can cause considerable discomfort, it is better to avoid treating patients with minor liver damage and concentrate on those with aggressive disease. They argue that patients with mild disease are unlikely to develop significant complications in the near future, and as new, better, treatments are discovered, it is likely that, before those with mild disease deteriorate significantly, different drugs with fewer side-effects will be available.

On the other hand, some hepatologists feel that the mere presence of the virus is enough to warrant therapy and they recommend treating all patients with HCV. Their aim is to avoid any risk of later damage to the liver and to reduce the possibility of the virus being passed on.

The clinical goal of treatment is to clear the virus from the patient's system permanently so that the liver functions normally and damage caused by the virus heals. Evidence of success is threefold:

• normal LFTs,
• PCR negative,
• improved liver biopsy results.

(See Chapter 2 for descriptions of these tests.)

What is Interferon?

'Interferon' is a generic term for a family of proteins that the body produces to ward off viral infections. Whenever you get a cold or flu your body makes large amounts of interferon, and this natural substance helps to kill the virus. In the process of attacking the virus, natural interferon makes you feel ill. When you have flu, for example, many of the symptoms, such as high fever, headaches, joint pains, are the result of interferon, not of the virus. In a similar way, when patients are treated with manufactured interferon they experience side-effects that are reminiscent of flu symptoms.

Many people wonder why a natural compound like interferon should be associated with such disagreeable side-effects. It is worth noting that it is the symptoms of viral illness that prevent you going out and passing the virus on to others. In other words, the side-effects, although unpleasant for the patient, serve to protect other members of the community.

In patients with chronic HCV, natural interferon, that is, the substance produced by your own body to help you fight infection, is not made in sufficient quantities to ward off the virus. The idea behind treatment is that by giving you huge amounts of synthetic interferon, your bodily defences become so fortified that your system eliminates the virus.

Interferon has three therapeutic properties:

- *antiviral powers* – it attacks and destroys the virus;
- *immune modulation* – it beefs up the immune system so that it can recognize and neutralize cells that are infected by the virus;
- *antiproliferation* – it slows down or halts the proliferation of some cancer cells.

The third of these properties has led to interferon being used to treat patients with cancer, and indeed it is an effective treatment for some, but by no means all, tumours. It is possible that interferon treatment may help to prevent primary liver cancer in patients with hepatitis C.

Interferon Therapy

The first drug used to treat hepatitis C was interferon alpha. This is given by injection into the skin, usually three times a week, for at least a year. With interferon monotherapy, that is, taking interferon alone, only one person in four remains free of the virus when treatment is stopped. People who take a course of interferon fall into three categories:

- *Non-Responders*   Approximately 50 per cent of patients who are treated with interferon shows no response at all. The virus continues to damage the liver and the LFTs (liver function tests) show no material improvement. These patients are called 'non-responders'. Patients, who have shown no response to interferon therapy after three months will not benefit from further treatment, and the drug is usually stopped.
- It is difficult to give up treatment when you have psyched yourself up for a year of it and gone through several weeks of injections and side-effects only to find that the drug has not worked. You should console yourself with the fact that you have given the treatment your best shot, and that new drugs are under investigation, which may allow you to receive more successful therapy in the future.
- *Relapsers*   The other 50 per cent of patients who receive interferon show an early response to treatment. The virus disappears from the blood and, after three months of therapy, the LFTs return to normal. Unfortunately half the number of patients who show an early response subsequently relapse, that is, the virus comes back, either during the treatment or soon after the interferon has been stopped. These patients are called 'relapsers' and it is disappointing to see that the virus has returned and that the liver has once again become inflamed.

- If you relapse during or after interferon you may receive comfort from the fact that for a period of time your liver functioned normally and the virus was under control. This means that your liver had a chance to regain some of its strength and the treatment probably slowed down the deterioration of your liver. Many patients who relapse after treatment are keen to try treatment with interferon again. This is not usually recommended, as a second course of interferon tends to be unsuccessful.
- *Complete Responders* 20 to 25 per cent of treated patients clear the virus, so that six months after treatment the virus cannot be detected and the LFTs are normal. These patients are called 'complete' or 'sustained' responders. It is rare for the virus to return after a complete response to interferon, and most people believe that patients who have responded completely to interferon are cured.
- However, interferon has been used to treat hepatitis C for only the last eight years or so. Although doctors can be sure that most patients who have had a complete response to interferon will be free of the virus for this length of time, they can not be absolutely certain that it never returns.

Combination Therapy for Hepatitis C

The relatively poor success rates with interferon mono-therapy led many doctors and scientists to develop other drugs that could be used in combination with interferon to improve the response rates. For many chronic infections, such as HIV and tuberculosis, using a number of different drugs simultaneously improves success rates.

The first drug to be tried in combination with interferon was ribavirin, which has been used for many years to treat a variety of viral infections. Pilot studies and recent trials have shown that adding ribavirin to interferon improves the long-term response rates to treatment. Many doctors now prescribe interferon plus ribavirin as the first-line treatment for hepatitis C.

Interferon and Ribavirin Treatment

The combination of interferon, which is injected three times a week, and ribavirin, which is taken in tablet form twice a day, gives you a 40 per cent chance of eliminating the virus and so effectively achieving a cure. Treatment lasts for six or twelve months, depending on which strain of HCV you are infected with. If you have HCV of genotype 1, your doctor will recommend twelve months of therapy, since shorter treatments are not as effective (for more information on genotypes see Chapter 1). If you have one of the other types of hepatitis C, genotypes 2 or 3, then you will need treatment for only six months, since prolonging treatment does not increase your chances of success.

As with interferon therapy on its own, some patients respond completely to interferon and ribavirin treatment, others respond initially and then relapse, while others do not respond at all. However, there is a very big difference in the time taken to respond to treatment. With interferon monotherapy everyone that responds shows early improvement in their LFTs, and the virus disappears within three months. The response to interferon plus ribavirin tends to be much slower.

If you receive interferon plus ribavirin, you should not be disappointed if your blood tests show no change during the first few months. Many patients who did not respond for up to six months have gone on to eliminate the virus completely.

Facts about Treatment

The current recommended course of interferon alone is three doses a week of three to six mega-units of interferon, usually for twelve months. Most doctors do not normally use interferon monotherapy but there are certain circumstances in which this is the most appropriate treatment. Ribavirin has a number of side-effects including iron deposition in the liver and breakdown of red blood cells. If your doctor is concerned that you may suffer as a result of these side-effects, he or she may recommend that you try interferon alone for a few months before considering combination treatment. You should discuss these issues with your clinician before embarking upon therapy.

Most patients start treatment with a combination of interferon and ribavirin. The ribavirin is given as capsules, usually four to six per day depending on body size. The interferon is given by injection three times a week. Each dose is injected into the skin above the stomach or into the thigh. The injection sites can be used in rotation.

Many balk at the prospect of injecting themselves. When Richard began his course of treatment, he was terrified:

'I couldn't believe it when the sister said I had to inject the medication. I had always been frightened of needles and the whole thing seemed desperate. How could my life have reduced to the level where I needed to stick sharp steel into my legs in order to preserve it?

'After the first injection, which the sister gave to me, I fainted. I was frightened of being hurt and of what the drugs might do to me.

'With the help of my fiancée, I began practising with the hypodermics and built up enough confidence to do the injections by myself. Within a few weeks, I was able to do them on my own without panicking. I often used to shudder when it was time for the next dose, but I managed to take the medicine all the same.'

The clinic you attend will show you how to perform the injections and a nurse will give you the first one or two. It may be useful to ask a friend, partner or relative to help. For example, Luca, a nervous Italian patient, got his mother to inject him instead of doing it himself. Like Richard, most patients find that they get accustomed to administering the injections, once they work through their initial fear.

Side-effects

The reported side–effects of taking interferon or interferon plus ribavirin are considerable. They are most pronounced at the start of treatment and generally become better tolerated over time. The important thing to remember is that there is a wide range of side-effects and a spectrum of responses to each. It is likely that you will have some, but not all, with varying degrees of intensity.

Common early side-effects are:

- flu-like symptoms, including hot and cold chills, muscle aches and pains, dry mouth, dehydration and headaches,
- poor appetite,
- tiredness,
- irritability.

Common late side-effects are:

- hair loss,
- weight loss,
- dry or itchy skin,

- pain at the sites of injection,
- loss of sex drive,
- lowering of sperm count,
- depression, anxiety, irritability and a predisposition to weep.

Occasionally, other side-effects occur, such as:

- seizures,
- thyroid disease,
- severe bone marrow suppression, reduction of white blood cells,
- acute psychosis, suicidal depression.

For most patients the side-effects reverse themselves within a few weeks of the end of the course of therapy, although treatment of a persistent side-effect is sometimes required.

Ribavirin usually intensifies the side-effects of interferon. In addition, there are some problems that are specific to ribavirin:

- *Haemolytic anaemia* Ribavirin causes the red blood cells to break down, which can lead to what is usually mild haemolytic anaemia. Sometimes the number of red blood cells falls to such a level that people become extremely tired. This condition generally improves when the dose of ribavirin is reduced, but occasionally the drug has to be stopped. If this happens, then you may want to continue with interferon alone to see whether you can eliminate the virus.
- *Effects on foetuses* Doctors know from experiments in animals that if ribavirin is present in the body when a baby is conceived, serious birth defects can occur. It is abso-

lutely vital that women taking ribavirin do not become pregnant. It is also important that women do not get pregnant until at least one year after treatment has finished, as the drug lingers in your system for a long time.

- *Effects on men's sperm*   Ribavirin may damage sperm. It is crucial that men taking ribavirin do not father children during treatment and for up to one year after treatment has finished.

You will appreciate that effective contraceptive measures are necessary while you are taking ribavirin, and that these measures should be continued for at least a year after treatment has ceased.

Future Parenthood and Interferon/Ribavirin

An area of particular concern relating to therapy is that of future parenthood. Both sexes face a potential problem. For a woman there is a timing dilemma, while for a man there is the worry about the effect of the drug on his sperm.

The female predicament   Interferon and ribavirin are toxic and therefore potentially dangerous to unborn babies. The effects of interferon on pregnant humans is unknown. In some animals interferon given during pregnancy has no harmful effects, but in other species interferon damages the unborn offspring. Ribavirin is harmful to unborn babies.

Because the risks to human babies are not fully known, interferon should not be given to pregnant women. It is also strongly urged that women of childbearing age should use an effective contraceptive while taking interferon. You must not conceive while on ribavirin or for twelve months following its use.

If you are being treated and become pregnant, then it is

imperative that you stop treatment immediately and contact your doctor. Special scans can be arranged to help decide whether the treatment has harmed your baby. You can then discuss whether it is wise to continue with the pregnancy.

Women with chronic hepatitis in their mid- to late thirties, who want to conceive, face a hard choice in deciding whether or not to be treated. If you are in this predicament, then you must resolve the following dilemma:

- *Horn 1*: Every year after you are 35 it becomes more difficult to have a baby, until by the time you are 42 and over conception is unlikely. Treatment for HCV lasts a year, and you must not conceive for up to a year after it has been completed. If you undergo drug therapy now, you may be too old to have a baby when you finish.
- *Horn 2*: It might be that it takes you a year or two to become pregnant because your biological clock is ticking away and your fecundity is diminishing. The longer you delay treatment, the more time the virus has to damage your liver and the more difficult it becomes for you to defeat it. If you have your baby first and then treat your disease, you may have ruined your chances of clearing the virus. In addition, you will be feeling the side-effects of the interferon just when you need all your strength to look after a young child. Finally, there is a small possibility of transmitting the infection to your baby.

The male predicament Interferon tends to lower a man's sperm count. Usually, this side-effect reverses after treatment stops. Men with normal sperm counts before they receive drug therapy are not believed to have a problem. Men with low sperm counts should seek expert advice in case the drug therapy does permanent damage to their fertility. Men who take ribavirin will need to wait until a year after their treatment before fathering children.

How to Make a Decision about Treatment

Taking interferon alone or interferon plus ribavirin is a serious matter. At the very least you can expect to feel ill during the first few weeks and inconvenienced for the rest of the treatment period. You need to reach a reasoned decision on whether you want treatment, if you are offered it. While every patient's individual circumstances and experience of the illness are unique, it is helpful to bear in mind the following general matters.

Points in Favour of Treatment
- You have a 40 per cent chance of clearing the virus in the long-term and so achieving a permanent cure.
- You have a further 25 per cent chance of clearing the virus during treatment and so giving your liver a much needed rest from inflammation.
- Even if you do not clear the virus, you may shift from having aggressive to mild disease.
- You may experience only mild and temporary side-effects, in which case being treated will cause minimal discomfort.

Points Against Treatment
- Not everybody treated is a complete responder.
- Interferon has to be given by injection.
- There are temporary but unpleasant side-effects.
- You will probably need to take a few weeks off work at the start of treatment.
- You may feel ill or at least under the weather for the duration of therapy.
- You may have to delay starting a family.
- New, better drugs may be available in the future that will eradicate the virus without the inconvenience and side-effects of current treatments.

Anyone with a history of mental illness needs to take special care because interferon can exacerbate any psychiatric disorder. Most doctors will not consider treating patients with a previous history of mental problems because the risk of a breakdown is too high. Discussion with the specialist is vital on this point.

Once you have gathered all the medical information, you must weigh up in your own mind whether you want treatment. Ask people who have undergone therapy what it was like for them. Attend support groups and find out what their members think. Discuss the issue with your friends, family and partner. Most importantly, find out what your doctor thinks about you receiving treatment and about how you will cope.

Preparation for Treatment

If you decide to go through with treatment, it is helpful to plan ahead. Prepare yourself for the worst, although with luck your experience will fall far short of it:

- Assume two weeks of housebound incapacity for the initial period of treatment.
- Take time off routine life: no work, no social commitments, etc..
- Stock up on food and soft drinks.
- Make sure your friends, family and support group contacts know what you are up to, because you will need their help.
- Pay your utilities bills: you do not want your phone or gas cut off when you are least able to think straight.
- Make sure your television and radio work and have a few good books and magazines to hand.
- Expect some immediate side-effects: fever, pain in the

gums, strange sensations in muscles and bones, aches and pains, and dehydration.
• Keep the clinic's emergency number by your telephone in case you have to contact the doctor or nurse.

The Experience of Treatment

People on drug therapy experience the side-effects in many different ways. Some find the treatment so debilitating that they have to stop – they are just too tired, depressed or sick to continue. Others have particular complications such as the significant loss of white blood cells, in which case the doctor advises them to give up treatment since the harm it is causing exceeds its potential benefits. The majority tolerate the side effects very well.

Jamie, 38, a sex therapist from Camden Town, found the whole thing gruelling, but persevered all the same:

'Taking interferon was the most disgusting experience of my life. I was depressed and amotivated and felt sick. I had permanent flu symptoms for the six months I was on interferon. I felt like an 80-year-old man.'

At the other end of the spectrum, some people feel only minimal discomfort, and go about their daily routine with virtually no interruption. Ian, an architect from Chelsea, continued his life much as normal:

'I began with doses of five mega-units of interferon for six months and then continued with three mega-units for another half year. During the first week I felt very tired and slightly sick. I had a couple of days off work to see how the injections affected me.

'To my surprise I was able to go back to work within a week

and be fairly productive. On the downside, my concentration was reduced and I felt irritable. I kept getting annoyed with my secretary without knowing why. Soon I became more relaxed and my temper was less frayed.

'Generally speaking, I felt tired for about eighteen hours after I had taken an injection. By lunchtime the following day I was almost back to normal.

'During the twelve months of treatment I took off two or three days from work, apart from at the outset, which were entirely due to the interferon. Of course, I was going to bed earlier than usual, but otherwise my routine was unchanged.'

Your experience of treatment is likely to fall somewhere in between those of Jamie and Ian. You can reasonably expect to feel tired, irritable and occasionally depressed, after you have passed through the induction period. Your concentration will be diminished, but not wiped out.

Monitoring and Motivation

From the clinical point of view, it is necessary to monitor patients on drug therapy carefully. You will be given frequent blood tests to check for abnormalities and to see if you are responding.

It is satisfying to learn that the abnormalities in your LFTs are reducing as a consequence of the medication. Richard found this motivated him:

'When I started on interferon I felt horrible and wondered whether the suffering was worth it. When I got my first blood test results, my ALT had dropped from 165 to 91 after only two weeks. By week six of treatment my ALT was within normal range.

'I was ecstatic. For the first time in twenty or more years, my liver was functioning properly. I was spurred on to take the medication when I realized that it was doing me some good.'

You need to bear in mind, though, that waiting for and hearing blood test results can be a hell as well as a heaven. Finding out that you have not fully responded or that you have relapsed can lead to despair. This may cause you to be extra anxious about the next blood test in case this confirms the bad news.

The secret is to live one blood test at a time. Do not predict what the results are going to be. When you are told what they are, discuss their significance with your doctor. Do not panic. Acknowledge any feelings of disappointment or outrage, but cultivate an optimistic outlook. You need hope as your weapon against despair.

Finishing Treatment

Determining when to complete treatment is a clinical decision made by your doctor with your input. A standard course of treatment lasts six months to a year. What you need to understand is the significance of your particular response. Your doctor can tell you how you have been getting on physiologically, so far as your blood tests reveal this. Only you can tell how the treatment affects you psychologically.

The moment will arrive when you stop treatment. Without fail, you will feel great relief. On finishing his medication, William's depression, induced by the drugs, evaporated:

'During treatment I felt as if a theatre curtain had fallen on me and wrapped itself around me. I seem to weigh tons and tons and only had black thoughts.

'When I finished my treatment, it was as though the huge leaden wrapper had been removed. I was capable of enjoying myself after being depressed for a long time. I was glad to be normal again.'

Prognosis for Responders

The future looks bright for complete responders. If your LFTs are normal and your PCR is negative six months after the end of treatment, then it is very likely that your liver has healed and you will stay free of hepatic infection. Studies indicate that those who sustain their response for a number of years suffer no further damage to their livers, except in a small number of cases where cirrhosis has progressed beyond the point of control. There are many cases where badly damaged livers have gone back to a totally healthy state.

If you maintain your response, then the symptoms of your viral infection will no longer trouble you. You will become stronger over time and will not suffer from hepatic fatigue, nausea and malaise. All the same, it is advisable to continue managing your lifestyle so that you remain in good shape.

It is not yet known whether the virus can return after, say, five or six years of remission. Even if it does, it is unlikely to have much power. If you are lucky enough to clear the virus through therapy, then you are effectively cured.

Re-treatments and Maintenance Therapies

For patients who have received a course of interferon and failed to respond at all, that is, non-responders, there is currently no further available therapy. Very little is gained by taking a course of interferon and ribavirin, since the chances of responding successfully are very small. Similarly, patients who have failed to respond to interferon and ribavirin are unlikely to respond to therapies that are other available. However, new drugs against HCV are being developed all the time and it is likely that new, improved therapies will be on offer in the near future.

For relapsers to interferon monotherapy, that is, patients who were PCR-negative during treatment, but who become positive again afterwards, there is the possibility of re-treatment with interferon and ribavirin. Indeed, it appears that people who showed a partial response to an initial course of interferon have a very good chance of responding to combination therapy. Many doctors are now offering combination therapy to patients who had a partial response to an initial course of therapy.

Some individuals are 'interferon dependent', that is, they become free of the virus and have normal LFTs whenever they are on medication, but lose their response as soon as the drugs are withdrawn. Such patients may be kept on a part time regime of treatment. For example, they may have six months on medication and six months off.

In very exceptional cases, a maintenance programme is required. Only those with multiple infections or cirrhosis, or who are very young, are likely to be offered such therapy.

Amantadine

'Amantadine' is an antiviral tablet that has been used for many years to treat people with serious influenza. It is also widely used for the treatment of a brain disorder called Parkinson's disease, where it stimulates the abnormal brain in a positive manner. A few studies have looked at the combination of interferon and amantadine in patients with chronic hepatitis C. It appears that amantadine makes interferon more effective and, surprisingly, reduces the side-effects of interferon, thereby making treatment more palatable.

The full effects of amantadine in patients with hepatitis C are currently under investigation and doctors do not yet know whether interferon and amantadine will be as effective as the combination of interferon and ribavirin. The results of this research will be available within the next year or so. At the moment amantadine is only used by patients who are enrolled on clinical trials.

Pegylated Interferon

A new species of interferon, called 'pegylated interferon', has reached the trial stage in the treatment of hepatitis C. Two problems with interferon are the need for it to be injected three times a week and the speed with which it dissipates through a patient's system. The relapse rate for patients on interferon has been high and a suspicion is that this results from its rapid elimination.

Pegylated interferon is interferon that is chemically linked to another molecule (poly-ethylene glycol – PEG), which extends its half-life. As a result it disperses through the body at a much slower rate than interferon and hammers the virus for a more protracted time. It is hoped that pegylated interferon will clear the virus in many more cases than does ordinary interferon. A material benefit is that it needs to be administered only once a week, and therefore causes minimal patient distress.

Other Drugs in the Pipeline

A lot of research into cures for hepatitis C is going on, and medical scientists are confident that something highly effective for treating most patients with chronic disease will be discovered in the near future. Among potential treatments under investigation are new interferons, urso-deoxycholic acid, non-steroidal anti-inflammatory agents, N-acetyl L-cysteine, iron depletion, and a combination of interferon and thymosin. Although improvement in LFTs has resulted from trials of some of these therapies, the long-term effects are not yet known.

If you are a non-responder or a relapser, you can be confident that new and better treatments will become available. So long as you are not in immediate danger from your virus, you have little to fear as you will receive the rewards of advancing medical science in the foresee-able future.

Clinical Trials

As new drugs are developed, it is important that they are properly tested on volunteer patients to decide whether they are likely to be helpful or not. There are two basic types of clinical trials: *controlled clinical trials* and *dose-finding studies*.

Controlled clinical trials are trials designed to find out whether a new treatment actually works or not. A large number of patient volunteers will be randomly allocated to treatment with either a new drug or an existing drug (usually interferon in the case of treating hepatitis C). Patients are not allowed to choose which treatment they receive, since this would bias the trial – all the enthusiastic patients would take the new drug and all the conservative patients would opt for the old drug.

After random allocation to one treatment or the other, patients are dosed with their drug for a certain amount of time, and all the patients' responses are carefully monitored. At the end of the trial, the numbers of patients who have benefited in each group are compared with those who have not, and the likelihood of success in the future treatment of patients is calculated.

It is standard practice for trials to include an extension clause that allows non-responding patients to receive the best treatment at the end of the trial, if they did not receive it during the trial. In other words, if drug X was compared to interferon and was shown to be the more effective of the two, all the patients who had received interferon and not responded would be offered drug X at the end of the study.

Dose-finding studies are short trials in which a new drug is given to a few patients to decide what is the most effective dose. These studies are undertaken simply to work out what is the best dose of a drug to use.

If you have the opportunity to take part in a clinical trial, you should weigh up the pros and cons carefully before making your decision.

Advantages of taking part in a trial   You may receive a new drug much sooner than would otherwise be possible. New drugs are normally not available for several years after they have been developed. It takes time to license a drug and to build facilities for its production. It is often only possible to obtain a new drug as part of a clinical trial. Also, you are contributing to medical knowledge about hepatitis C and playing a significant role in finding better treatments.

Disadvantages of taking part in a trial   You will be receiving a new drug whose side-effects are unknown or incompletely known. All drugs are tested as much as they can be before they are given to patients, but nevertheless unexpected problems do occasionally occur. It is not always possible to predict the side-effects associated with new drugs. Second, you will have to attend the clinic or hospital regularly, perhaps quite frequently: clinical trials often involve extra visits and blood tests, since it is important to pay special attention to the effect of the new drug on you.

Before agreeing to take part in a clinical trial, you should think carefully about what you are letting yourself in for. You should discuss what it involves with your hepatologist and make sure that you have all the information necessary to make a prudent decision. Remember that if you decide not to participate in a trial, your treatment will not be affected by your decision. Your doctor will continue to look after you in exactly the same way as before.

Conclusion

Treatment with prescribed drugs is a risk. You may become depressed. You may hate doing the injections. It may not work. But the potential reward is fabulous: you can clear the virus and have no further trouble from chronic hepatitis C. To all intents and purposes you can be cured.

Those who do not respond fully need not give up hope. There are various alternative strategies on offer and new treatments are constantly entering the trial stage.

A further reward of undergoing treatment, should you so decide, is that you do something loving for yourself. Whether it is successful or not, you can give it your best shot and know with much satisfaction that you are doing all you can.

6

Western Complementary Medicine

People make use of complementary medicine for many reasons. Some turn to it after conventional medicine has failed to cure them. Naturopaths believe that it offers the only acceptable form of treatment, regarding drug therapy as too harmful to the individual.

There is also a view which holds that both conventional and complementary medicine have something to offer. Those who take this approach accept that complementary therapies may have a role to play in lifestyle management, while also taking seriously the possibility of drug treatment to clear the virus.

It is crucial to understand the problems associated with complementary medicine, as well as its potential. Once you are aware of them, you can take sensible steps both to minimize any potential risks and to maximize your chances of deriving benefit.

What is Complementary Medicine?

'Complementary medicine' is an umbrella term referring to many forms of treatment. There are two main branches: western complementary medicine (WCM) and traditional

Chinese medicine. Homoeopathy, supplements, certain herbs, superfood and massage are examples of western complementary medicine and are covered in this chapter; acupuncture and Chinese herbs are examples of the eastern variety, which we look at in Chapter 7.

It is important to understand that conventional medicine and WCM proceed on completely different bases.

Conventional medicine is founded on scientific method. This means that its treatments are tested under laboratory conditions and subjected to rigorous scrutiny. The aim is to form a rational and balanced picture of whatever treatment is under review. For instance, before a drug is licensed (that is, approved by the government for public use) it is thoroughly analysed in clinical trials and its dangers recorded and made known, where possible.

WCM does not operate in this way. Remedies are tried and adopted if they are successful. What counts as 'successful' is not always what science understands by this term. In general, no detailed analysis of how or why something works is, or often can be, given by practitioners of WCM.

Cynics hold that WCM has only a 'placebo effect' – that is, it makes you feel good because you have taken something. It is certainly true that doing something helpful for yourself gives you a psychological boost. However, it may not be the case that this is all that WCM provides. As yet, no one fully understands what it does, and this leaves open the question as to its benefits.

Doctors and Complementary Medicine

Most conventional doctors are sceptical about complementary medicine. This doubt is based on several problems associated with alternative treatments, some applicable in general, some related in particular to treating liver disease.

Lack of Proper Regulation

Conventional doctors have to undergo a set period of training and, once qualified, they have to maintain certain standards; if they do not, they can be barred from practising. By contrast, anyone can set him- or herself up as a complementary medical practitioner and treat patients. There is no legal requirement to obtain any qualifications, nor is there any professional obligation to maintain a patient's confidentiality. Of course, recognized, genuine practitioners of complementary medicine are just as concerned as conventional doctors about unqualified practitioners and many have set up their own working groups with appropriate controls to prevent abuse.

Lack of Evidence of Success

There is no hard evidence that complementary medicine actually works. Conventional drugs are tested in controlled conditions to discover precisely what proportion of patients taking the treatment will benefit and what proportion will suffer harm from side-effects. This information is published and is available to the general public. No such data exist for complementary medicine.

Those working in the field claim that because complementary medicine diagnoses every patient on an individual basis, no comparison can be drawn between the treatments used in different cases. This argument may well have its merits, but it makes it difficult to validate the benefits claimed for complementary medicine.

Special Dangers for Liver Complaints

Some herbs and compounds used in complementary medicine for liver complaints can have harmful side-effects. For example, the Jamaican herb 'bush tea' is well recognized as a cause of scarring of the liver. Some herbs have even been associated with fulminant hepatitis and death from liver failure.

It is quite wrong to claim that because a product is 'natural' it cannot have side-effects. You should recall that hemlock is a natural product and that interferon, although now produced by genetic engineering, is based on a natural compound.

Deciding Whether to Use WCM

If you are thinking of having a WCM treatment, it is essential to be fully informed of what it entails before making a decision. Being wise after the event will not protect your health. The authors are not aware of anyone who has been cured by complementary medicine.

- Read all the literature you can find on the subject. Most reputable WCM bodies will have a number of relevant pamphlets or can suggest other reading on the treatments that they offer.
- Speak to any friends or acquaintances who have used complementary remedies. They may be able to endorse a form of treatment or practitioner that they have found helpful, or sound a note of warning about a less pleasant experience.
- Make sure that you consult a certified practitioner. There are registers of those who are authorized to offer complementary treatments. Ask to see the practitioner's qualifications and certificates. Ask the practitioner how long he or she has been practising.
- Find out whether the practitioner has liability insurance. Reputable practitioners, like all conventional doctors, are insured to protect themselves from litigation in the event that any patient develops problems associated with his or her treatment. If your practitioner does not have insurance you must ask yourself why not. If a professional insurance company regards this practitioner as likely to

cost them large sums of money in damages, do you really want to entrust your health to this person?

- Ask the practitioner why he or she proposes a particular treatment and what the expected benefits and side-effects are. You should be very sceptical about extravagant claims. There is no magical cure for HCV. Your practitioner may be able to help you with some of your symptoms and may help you in coming to terms with your illness, but claims of a guaranteed cure are likely to be false.
- Discuss the recommended treatment with your liver specialist and members of your support group (if you attend one) before undergoing it. They may be able to affirm its value or warn you of any dangers.

Remember the reservations about WCM:

- The effects of remedies are often unpredictable, as no one really knows how these things work.
- The benefits are not usually proven.
- Expectations of a cure can be raised and then dashed.
- Treatments can be expensive (see section below on 'The Costs of WCM').

The Importance of Not Self-Prescribing
If you are coming into contact with WCM for the first time, you might be tempted to prescribe things for yourself. You might read about, say, milk thistle in this book and then start taking tons of it without consulting a practitioner. *Don't.*

You may not get the proper benefit that something might produce for you. You might take too much or too little, or take the remedy the wrong way or at the wrong time. A further concern is that some complementary products can be harmful and so need professional prescription, even if you can buy them over the counter.

The Holistic Approach

WCM adopts a holistic approach to medicine. This means that the whole person – mind, body and spirit – is taken into account in determining an appropriate course of action. Conventional medicine, by contrast, tends to concentrate treatment on a specific symptom or complaint. For example, if you have constipation, then a laxative may be prescribed. In WCM a complete picture of the patient's background, symptoms and mental states is considered relevant to the diagnosis. Consequently, at your first few appointments with a WCM practitioner, a detailed record of certain facts about you will be required. Some of the questions which are asked may well seem irrelevant to the condition for which you are seeking relief. Do not be put off by having to give a biography of yourself!

Homoeopathy

Homoeopathy was developed by a conventional doctor called Samuel Hahnemann over 300 years ago as a method of treatment whereby the body's natural capacity to heal itself is intensified. It involves the administration (usually in extremely diluted form) of substances that in a healthy person would produce symptoms similar to those of the complaint being treated.

It assumes that symptoms represent disharmony within the whole person and that it is the patient, rather than the disease, that requires treatment. The homoeopath interviews the patient in detail about his or her medical history, family background and general state of mind as well as the particular symptoms.

Homoeopathic remedies are regarded as non-addictive and are claimed to have no side-effects. Occasionally there is a temporary aggravation of the condition that is being treated before it settles down and, it is hoped, improves.

Tony, a 45-year-old graphic designer from Brixton, has begun this form of treatment for his chronic hepatitis:

> 'Recently, I've started using homoeopathic cures. My wife put me in touch with a practitioner. I like the idea of using natural remedies to reinforce the body's ability to fight off disease. It doesn't use poisons like conventional medicine.
>
> 'When I saw the homoeopath, she talked to me about my hepatitis and my life which I described to her. She gave me some little white pills which I've begun to take. I don't know if I've had any positive effects yet because I've only just started with her.'

Vitamins, Minerals and Other Supplements

This category of WCM is the most studied and has won the greatest degree of acceptance by conventional medicine. A practitioner will prescribe a course of vitamins and other supplements, to be taken daily, with three purposes in mind:

- to strengthen the liver's capacity to rebuild itself;
- to boost the immune system;
- to attack any viruses that are present.

Vitamins and minerals are essential for health whatever condition you are in. If you suffer from a deficiency in any vitamin you will become unwell.

In affluent western societies a balanced diet generally provides more than enough vitamins and minerals to keep you healthy. Some practitioners believe that because adequate vitamins and minerals are necessary for normal health, an excess will provide extra benefits in cases of ill-health.

This sort of treatment requires a lot of commitment. You must follow the instructions carefully or you may not gain the maximum benefit. These instructions can be complicated, with many different doses to be taken at different – not always convenient – times of the day. Your shelves are likely to be stacked with bottles and plastic containers full of pills and capsules. Keeping track of them and making sure you replenish each sort before you run out can be a stock control nightmare.

The supplements that are commonly prescribed for hepatitis patients include the following.

Vitamin C

Vitamin C is an antioxidant – a substance that delays the process of deterioration by oxidation – and diminishes the activity of free radicals, which are certain atoms or groups of atoms that cause cellular damage.

A side-effect of taking too much of it is diarrhoea. The reason for this is that the body does not store vitamin C and tends to excrete excess amounts.

Vitamin B Complexes

The B vitamins are a large family of substances involved in the metabolism of all living cells. They work together with proteins in the various enzyme systems of the body. They have antioxidant powers similar to vitamin C and so may prevent damage to liver cells.

Zinc

Zinc is an important trace mineral, essential to the immune system. In patients with a zinc deficiency, wound healing is impaired. Occasionally, hepatitis patients are deficient in zinc, though the conditions are not linked.

Magnesium

About half of the magnesium in the body combines with calcium and phosphorus to strengthen the bones and teeth. The remainder is in the red blood cells, muscles and other soft tissue, where it reduces excess blood clotting. It is also needed in many enzyme systems, especially those involved with energy production.

In those hepatitis patients who are deficient in magnesium, supplements are required, and will be prescribed by conventional doctors.

N-Acetyl L-Cysteine

This is not a true vitamin but shares certain properties with some vitamins. It is an antioxidant, which scavenges free radicals and toxic oxygen by-products, thus protecting the liver, lungs and blood. It is used to treat various liver disorders because of its detoxifying function. It is used in conventional medicine in cases of fulminant hepatitis, where it is of proven benefit; but its effects in other liver disorders are unknown.

Western Herbs

Western herbs are frequently prescribed in conjunction with vitamins and other supplements. They have been an integral part of traditional folk medicine for over two thousand years. The following herbs are claimed to be of value to hepatitis sufferers.

Milk Thistle (Silymarin)

This herb is thought to be anti-inflammatory, to protect the liver from viral injury and to aid regeneration of healthy cells. It contains certain substances reputed to protect the liver, referred to collectively as silymarin. This is an antioxidant that suppresses the factors responsible for hepatic injury, namely free radicals and leukotrienes, which are damaging compounds that are usually destroyed by protective body mechanisms. It also stimulates protein synthesis, which boosts production of new liver cells to replace damaged old ones.

Conventional medicine recognizes some of the potential of silymarin and scientists in the United States and Germany have been researching it for over twenty years. In Germany it is sometimes prescribed for patients on interferon.

However, recent studies of patients with alcoholic liver disease have found no benefit from silymarin treatment.

In the first few days of treatment, silymarin may cause irritability, headache or stomach upset, but these side-effects subside in due course.

Liquorice Root
This is used as a primary ingredient in many herbal traditions for a variety of conditions, including viral hepatitis. It is considered to have a liver-protecting effect, although its mechanisms are different from those of milk thistle. It is an antioxidant and has direct antiviral properties. It may also stimulate interferon and antibody production. Trials in Japan have brought it to the attention of conventional medicine and some doctors consider it to be beneficial if administered within proper regimes.

Liquorice root is known to have considerable side-effects if taken in large doses or for a long time.

Dandelion Root
This is believed to cleanse the bloodstream, to increase the production of bile, and to reduce cholesterol and uric acid. It has been taken for cirrhosis, hepatitis, anaemia, cramps and fluid retention.

American Superfood

'Superfood' is a family name for products that contain blue-green algae, spirulina, chlorella, salina or other comparable substances. The raw materials are algae, which are harvested from lakes. The individual types can be taken on their own if so wished; the advantage of a packaged superfood is that the quantities and qualities of the ingredients are stated on the product label and thus are guaranteed.

Algae have been used as a food source for at least four thousand years, with the ancient Aztecs known to have relied on them as a staple. Kanembu tribesmen living near Lake Johann in Chad in the African Sahara desert still make and eat algae cakes. Today, superfood producers farm their algae on lakes in America and Australia. They freeze-dry their crops to preserve the natural contents and the resultant product usually comes in powder form.

The main advantage of superfood is that it contains a very high level of nutrients in a virtually pure and easily digestible form. Its fans among hepatitis patients claim that it:

- boosts energy;
- strengthens the immune system;
- places no strain on the liver;
- increases mental alertness and stamina;
- rejuvenates short- and long-term memory.

Nicola, 36, a fine art restorer from Brompton, London, has achieved higher levels of physical and mental energy as a result of taking superfood. She was drawn to WCM because it addresses her as a whole person:

'The point of WCM is to treat the core rather than the surface. For example, conventional medicine treats a headache by giving you a pill to take away the pain. It doesn't necessarily help heal the problem, which usually extends beyond its felt presence.

'WCM deals with the person as a whole being, taking into account body, mind and spirit. I have found that this approach has been very helpful to me.

'One of the things I do is to take chlorella, which comes in capsules. At the moment I'm taking about thirty a day. I find that it cleanses out my system and lifts my energy. It's extremely high in protein and, being a vegetarian, it is a welcome kind of food.

'The person I know who inspired me to investigate it is a flute player who became paralysed as a result of aluminium poisoning. I have seen him get better over time and now he is completely healed as a result of taking chlorella.

'I believe that because it worked for him when nothing else did, it might work for me even though we have different complaints.'

Massage

Who said it wasn't any fun being ill? You need to relax, and massage assists this end as well as having therapeutic properties of its own.

During a massage an expert will pummel and pressurize different parts of your body surface in a way that most people find highly pleasurable. You have to be undressed for this form of treatment, although you wrap a towel around your waist and front, as required.

The specific aims of massage for the hepatitis patient are to:

- *De-stress* by toning up the muscles and improving the circulatory system;
- *Detoxify* by employing a technique called manual lymph drainage (MLD).

MLD is a special form of massage that concentrates on the lymphatic system, which is a network of capillary vessels that transports the fluid of the body as lymph, that is, in the form largely of white cells, to the blood circulation in the veins. Supporters of MLD claim that there are areas of the body where the muscles are stiff and the blood does not circulate freely. It is claimed that toxins get trapped in the muscles in these areas, and massage is supposed to release these pockets of toxins back into the system so that they can be flushed out properly.

The Costs of WCM

The cost of WCM is generally high. Each kind of treatment has its own fee structure, although as a general rule the first consultation is more expensive than later sessions, since it involves a long interview. In some areas of the country, limited public funds are available for certain treatments, in particular homoeopathy.

The following is a guide to the prices of the various treatments at the beginning of 1999.

- *Homoeopathy*: An initial consultation is £30–45, with subsequent appointments at £25–30. You may need to go once a month for the first year.
- *Vitamins, minerals and other supplements*: The initial and follow-up consultations cost about the same as for homoeopathy, but you will only need to go for three or four visits in the first year. The daily cost of the supplements will depend on what you are recommended. If you take a lot of them it can amount to £1–2 per day. It is sometimes cheaper to buy your supplies through a postal service than directly from a shop.
- *Western herbs*: The initial consultation fee is included in the

cost of the various herbs. They range in price depending on what you need, but expect to pay the same as for vitamins.

- *Superfood*: As a very rough guide, you should budget for £2–3 per day on superfood. You will notice that this is approximately the price of a takeaway meal from a junk-food restaurant, but with the possible advantage of enhancing your health.

- *Massage*: This costs £25–30 for the first session and then £20–25 for subsequent visits.

Conclusion

There are many types of western complementary treatments on offer to hepatitis C patients. Some have the approval of conventional medicine and others are unknown quantities. It is hoped scientific confirmation of the value of certain promising therapies will become available in the near future.

Many patients have enjoyed benefits from complementary remedies in terms of relieving some of their symptoms. If you are thinking of undergoing such a treatment, you must investigate the proposed course of action thoroughly before committing yourself to it, and you must be aware of the cost, which can be very high.

By keeping an open mind about WCM and possibly trying things that you feel could be helpful, you may do yourself a great service. There is certainly a therapeutic value at the psychological level in doing what you can to help yourself.

Some go further and maintain that there is actually a human need to ask for help, whether or not it produces the desired effect. The point is that should you ask for help in an honest and responsible manner, you are doing the best you can for yourself and showing faith, whatever the outcome of your efforts.

7

Traditional Chinese Medicine

The second branch of complementary medicine that is of interest to hepatitis patients is a number of treatments originating in the east. They comprise acupuncture, and the use of herbs, massage and exercise, as they have evolved within traditional Chinese medicine (TCM).

Although it is unfamiliar to most people in the west, TCM is gaining increased acceptance as sufferers begin to experience the fruits of this form of healing. Some claim not only that it can limit the progression of chronic disease, but that it can also clear the virus.

A Word of Warning

You should be aware that there are no properly substantiated reports of anyone being completely cured by TCM. There are, however, a few reported cases of patients suffering serious ill effects, and even dying, after taking Chinese herbal remedies. It is essential to consider the potential risks and benefits very carefully before undergoing TCM treatment.

The dilemma with TCM is how far to expect it to help. A conservative element within conventional medicine denies that it has any contribution to make, since many of the treatments have not yet been shown to be successful under laboratory conditions. On the other hand, more liberal minds see TCM as having positive value, at least in enhancing a person's sense of well-being.

You should bear in mind that TCM has no scientifically proven cure for hepatitis; very little research is done in the west with a view to validating TCM and controlled studies are rare. However, it does not follow that TCM *cannot* alleviate or cure hepatitis.

You should also recognize that while it may be alien for you to consider TCM, it is equally bizarre for a Chinese person to contemplate interferon therapy; yet you may think of drug treatment as perfectly justified. The unfamiliarity of a foreign system of healing need not be a barrier to its effectiveness.

It is interesting to note that certain mainstream liver specialists are beginning to investigate the potential benefits of some forms of TCM. Professor Batey of the John Hunter Hospital, New South Wales, Australia, has instigated a study to determine the effects of Chinese herbs on chronic viral infection. He is aware of the scepticism with which alternative remedies are viewed, but has attracted formal approval for his research all the same:

'The trial took an enormous amount of energy as most ethics committees are not used to endorsing the use of agents such as herbal products. Thirty-six patients have now been entered in the trial which will be evaluated after six months of treatment.

'Further studies will be undertaken should the herbal medicine preparation be shown to be efficacious. Already the organic chemistry department of a major university in Sydney has expressed interest in studying the product to determine what agents are likely to be active in inducing improvement in the disease process.'

Why You Might Consider TCM?

The main reason for trying TCM if you have viral hepatitis is that it might at least retard the progression of the disease. Bearing in mind the reservation that there is no proof of the success of its treatments according to western scientific criteria, a properly informed person may nevertheless judge that TCM is worth trying.

If you decide to undergo eastern complementary treatments, you must make sure that you tell your liver specialist what you intend to do. He or she can then monitor your progress or lack of it and help in judging its usefulness.

Christoff received only a modest improvement to his chronic condition from conventional medicine and turned to TCM as an alternative. He had taken interferon alone and undergone combination therapy of interferon and ribavirin, but his LFTs remained abnormal and the virus was still present. He thought that he would give Chinese herbs a chance:

'I decided I would try two years' alternative medicine before going back to the conventional approach. The specialist had said that I should undergo a re-treatment, but I wanted to try TCM first.

'Something about Chinese medicine appealed to me. They've been practising it for thousands of years. Having already had a course of chemotherapy, the thought of being treated naturally was very attractive. I was not going to have to inject all those drugs which seemed to poison my system.

'I had heard through a friend about a skilful Chinese

practitioner who had done well for someone with ME and someone else with an immune problem. Maybe he could help me with my hepatitis.

'I checked with the specialist at the liver unit and asked him if he thought I was mad to do this, and he said "No. We'll monitor you carefully and if we think it's harming you we'll tell you."'

Many hepatitis patients feel that they have benefited from TCM. They claim that the treatments have made them feel better and some even assert that the virus has been eradicated. It is important to remember that evidence of these cures is anecdotal.

The Theory Behind TCM

The only way to understand TCM is to put to one side all you know about conventional medicine. Because it is so different from what westerners are accustomed to, it can seem to have no rational foundation. The thing to bear in mind is that it has its own kind of justification, which, internal to itself, makes perfect sense. With an open mind, new and fruitful ideas can be taken on board and exciting treatments considered in their best light.

TCM works on the principle that a certain life force, called 'chi', operates within the body. When you have symptoms, chi is out of balance. The general aim of TCM is to restore the balance of chi by unblocking or damming up its effects according to various 'meridians' or imaginary lines passing through the body.

The life energy is described in terms of yin and yang. 'Yin' refers to what is cool, moist, deep, nourishing and still, 'yang' to what is warm, active and moving. Yin is on the inside, while yang is on the outside of the body. In ideal circumstances, the chi is kept moving so that the body is nourished from the inside by the yin energy and from the outside by the yang.

The TCM view of chronic hepatitis is that an infection is present to which the body reacts by creating a surplus of heat. This heat is welcome in the sense that it is an attempt by the body to ward off the infection; but it is damaging when it spreads out and dries up the yin – the cool, moist energy. This dehydrating process ultimately leads to the shrivelling of the liver – cirrhosis, as it is known in conventional medicine.

The kinds of questions TCM asks are: 'How hot is the body?' 'How moist is it?' 'How cold?' 'How dry?' 'How damp?' In response to the answers to these questions a practitioner treats the body in such a way as to keep it cool and to maintain its energy flow so that it is best able to sort itself out.

TCM recognizes that liver damage is often accompanied by bowel disorders. Hot liver energy invades the spleen, stomach and digestive system, resulting in upset, bloating, biliousness, diarrhoea or sometimes constipation. A state of 'damp heat' reigns, with damp caused by the impaired digestive system and heat spreading from the liver.

Liver conditions are revealed by examining the tongue. If the tongue is too red, then there is an excess of heat. If it is cracked, the yin is under pressure. The coating of the tongue tells the practitioner if toxins are present. Too much yellow or dryness and crusting indicate too much heat. An excess of wetness and greasiness suggest damp and heat together.

Acupuncture

Acupuncture is the best-known form of TCM. It is gaining widespread recognition in the western world. There are many practitioners available and some may be consulted through public health schemes.

An acupuncturist uses thin needles which are pushed into the skin at significant points. According to TCM, there is a network of energy lines running throughout the body. The practitioner diagnoses your problem by taking your pulse and inspecting your tongue and ear, and then determines which points on the energy grid need adjustment.

The needles are usually placed in the stomach, back and ear. When they are pushed in, tingling sensations occur. The experience tends to be pleasant and the first few sessions can induce euphoria and tiredness, as pent-up forces are released or restrained.

To date, acupuncture is the eastern treatment most easily tested by western criteria. When a needle is stuck into a point, a scientist can measure the resultant blood gases, respiratory rates, cardiac patterns and so on. It is generally thought to be a safe process in qualified hands.

Chinese Herbs

Although TCM does not recognize viruses in the same way as conventional medicine, it has been found that some Chinese herbs may be effective antiviral remedies. The objectives of a Chinese herbal treatment are to:

- counter the infection;
- clear waste toxins;
- soothe and nourish the liver;
- strengthen the spleen and stomach.

Herbs are prescribed in terms of certain formulae written in an anglicized version of Chinese. These pick out the appropriate quantities and types of herbs, which can be obtained from specialist dispensaries.

The prescriptions are presented in little packets, which you are required to brew into a thick tea. It can take forty minutes or more to produce a green liquid with what look like twigs sticking out of it. This is then cooled and drunk as laid down in the instructions (the 'twigs' are discarded).

Each set of formulae is unique, although there are many ingredients common to all mixtures given to hepatitis patients. It is both gratifying and worrying that no two sets are exactly the same: gratifying because the practitioner is treating your case on an individual basis, worrying because you do not have a precise precedent for your treatment.

For Christoff, his herbal remedy has produced appreciable results, of which his hospital has taken note:

'The treatment consists of taking herbal pills which are coated in liquorice morning and night, and then once a week I make up a soup of various tree barks, berries, ginseng and other stuff. I simmer all the ingredients in two litres of water for two hours and then drink what's left.

'To start with I felt odd after taking the herbs. I felt slightly under the weather. There were no immediate benefits.

'After a month I went back to the practitioner who was very interested in my tongue. There were some cuts at the back of it which were like dehydration cracking and he monitored those carefully. He said that there had been no change so far.

'Then, after about two months, I started to feel noticeably better. I had a lot more energy. I could get through the day and do a hard day's work. My eyes became clearer. Formerly, they had been muddy.

'I have found that I can cope with the demands of life

much better. I think this was due totally to the herbs because I haven't changed anything else.

'The results of my blood tests at the hospital have also improved. My ALT has stabilized to just outside normal range. I've still got viral activity, but it seems that the herbs have reduced the ferocity of my hepatitis. They have certainly made me feel well and enabled me to lead a fuller life.'

Be warned that there are recorded cases where Chinese herbs have aggravated liver damage. In particular, those with cirrhosis are vulnerable.

Reflexology

This is an ancient form of massage, which makes use of connections between the inner parts of the body and its extremities. It was practised in China as long ago as 3,000 BC and is thought to be one of the oldest kinds of natural healing.

In reflexology every organ and gland in the body is linked in some way to the soles of the feet or the palms of the hands. The places on the hands and feet where these connections end are known as reflex points. Any tenderness here signals weakness to the practitioner, who then applies pressure to them. The aim of the massage is to correct any imbalances in the ten zones of the body that this form of healing postulates and to free the flow of energy round the body.

Freeing the flow of energy may help the hepatitis patient by:

• revitalizing the body's capacity to heal itself and so offer protection against the onslaught from infection;

- decreasing tension that leads to stress;
- increasing blood flow, which assists in clearing away accumulated toxins, thereby reducing the workload of the liver. These toxins take the form of crystals made up of uric acid and calcium. They feel like grains of salt under the skin and gather around the joints. They can be broken down and ultimately flushed out of the system.

Shiatsu

Strictly speaking, shiatsu is a Japanese form of healing that makes use of the Chinese grid system of energy flow. It is a type of massage that is effectively acupuncture without the needles. It aims to relax the nervous system and to balance the physical functions of the body.

Shiatsu massage focuses on the hands and thumbs, with occasional diversions on to the knees or forearms. Pressure is applied to those points that the practitioner considers relevant to the patient's individual requirements. Nutritional guidance and specialized therapeutic exercises, designed to enhance the treatment, may sometimes be recommended in addition to the massage.

Chi Kung

This is a form of exercise and meditation intended to aid relaxation as well as to build up physical and mental strength. It is not like western forms of exercise, where the participant runs and jumps about or plays a ball game. 'Chi kung' means 'the study of the science of vital force through exercises and meditation'. It can take many years of practice to become a master of this art, but a few basic techniques, properly learned, can be enough to make a telling difference to your state of being. You will need to be taught a beginner's regime, whose purpose is to:

- arouse awareness of chi, which can bring about a sense of rejuvenation and vitality;
- circulate chi efficiently so that emotional and physical states are optimal;
- maximize the smooth functioning of the liver by preserving and enhancing positive body energy;
- reduce the pulsation in the heart and lungs to a more peaceful and relaxed state.

To the novice, doing chi kung exercises is like performing kung fu or karate in slow motion.

The Cost of TCM and Public Funding

Acupuncture, reflexology, shiatsu and chi kung each cost £35–40 for an initial consultation, somewhat less for each follow-up session. You may need to attend for up to a year, although exactly how long your course of treatment lasts depends on your individual circumstances. Chinese herbs can cost £1–2 each day depending on the prescription.

There is limited public funding for TCM. For example, patients in certain areas of London can be referred to the Gateway Clinic in Stockwell. This unit was established in 1988 and applies TCM to those with viral infections. At the outset it was mostly people with HIV who were treated, but growing numbers of hepatitis patients have been taken on.

This sort of pioneering work may blossom if it is successful. The hope is that TCM will become more widely available through public health schemes in the foreseeable future.

TCM and Hepatitis: A Summary

Chronic active hepatitis is understood and treated by TCM in its own unique way, which bears little resemblance to western equivalents.

According to TCM, the problem is that the free flow of chi and blood is impeded by the presence of infection. Excessive heat can:

- harm the yin energy of the body;
- infiltrate the pancreas and stomach, affecting digestion and the formation of chi and blood;
- dry the body fluid, blood and tissues of the liver.

The solution is to recreate balance throughout the body. This may be done in various ways:

- by acupuncture, to stimulate the circulation of chi and blood and to open the channels of the body to restore organic function;
- with Chinese herbs, to open, clear, nourish and strengthen the body;
- by reflexology and shiatsu, to move chi and blood and to unblock energy flow;
- by chi kung, to relax the mind and body and so enable the improved flow of chi.

Conclusion

Western science tends to be sceptical about the results of TCM, which are not proven. By the same token, its claims are not disproved. Thus, the question as to its efficacy remains open.

Some hepatitis C patients have enjoyed success with

TCM, when conventional medicine has not been able to help them. Others have used it as their first kind of treatment, either eschewing interferon therapy or just to see what it can do. At the very least a cosmetic benefit has been felt by some who have tried it.

The psychological reward of helping yourself to heal yourself is undeniable. Curiosity about something that is alien, yet potentially beneficial, shows not just an interest in the unknown, but a desire to get better at all costs. This kind of spirit may find you a cure in the most bizarre of places and against all the odds.

8

End-Stage Liver Disease and Transplants

Two ultimate perils threaten those with aggressive chronic hepatitis C: cancer and liver failure. In a few lucky cases, surgery can halt the decline; for the remainder, a degenerative process accelerates until the patient dies.

The symptoms of the final phase of the disease cycle are debilitating and quality of life spirals downwards. Hospitalization and long periods of being bedridden become commonplace.

Miraculously, technology is advancing to the point where there is a good chance of recovery from a transplant operation. Many people with advanced cirrhosis are given new livers and enjoy a full and active life.

Cancer

A grave danger associated with viral hepatitis is that of primary liver cancer, or 'hepatocellular carcinoma'. 'Primary' as opposed to 'secondary' disease means that the cancer originates in the liver rather than spreading there from somewhere else.

This kind of cancer amounts to the formation of one or

more tumours in the liver. The only treatment is localized surgery or a full transplant.

Patients with cirrhosis are most vulnerable to this problem. Every year a proportion of those with cirrhosis caused by HCV develop liver cancer. Survival rates are very low. However, if a tumour can be diagnosed while still in its early stages, the possibility of successful surgery is considerably increased.

Screening for Liver Cancer
Many liver units screen patients with HCV and cirrhosis, since they have a high risk of developing primary liver cancer. Symptoms that may indicate cancer – pain, loss of appetite, weight loss, lethargy, jaundice, ascites (swelling of the stomach) – usually develop only when the cancer is relatively large, and some of them may result from other, non-cancerous conditions. By performing regular blood and ultrasound tests, tumours can be detected at an early stage when treatment may be possible.

It is distressing to undergo regular screening for cancer. Simply attending for the test causes many patients considerable anxiety. You should reassure yourself that, in the vast majority of cases, the results will be normal. Furthermore, if an abnormality is discovered, then finding the tumour at an early stage will significantly improve your chances of a cure. So attending a clinic regularly, is a good precaution against any unwanted growths progressing too far. If you are unduly worried about how you feel between your scheduled visits, you should contact your specialist immediately so that additional investigation can be carried out.

Decompensated Cirrhosis

If you are unfortunate enough to have cirrhosis as a result of your viral infection, then you are in danger of progressing to the final stages of the hepatitis cycle. This is called 'end-stage liver disease' and consists of 'decompensated cirrhosis'.

Cirrhosis usually establishes itself without symptoms. There are few specific external markers to suggest what is going on inside the body. 'Compensated cirrhosis' is a condition in which the liver, although malfunctioning, performs its tasks well enough for normal life to continue.

If scarring and damage are allowed to proceed unhindered, the liver reaches a point where it can no longer provide the body with what it needs. It moves into a state of 'decompensated cirrhosis'. Effectively, the liver breaks down, like an old rusty car that cannot run any more.

At least 500 people in England and Wales, and over 3,000 in America, die of decompensated cirrhosis due to viral infection each year.

The Symptoms of End-Stage Liver Disease

A person in the last phase of the hepatitis cycle can expect to have some or all of the following symptoms:

Jaundice 'Jaundice' or going yellow is a common sign of decompensated cirrhosis. It is caused by the liver's loss of ability to remove bile pigment. The skin and eyes take on a yellow colour and the urine goes brown.

It is a common misconception that all liver diseases lead to jaundice. In fact, it affects only a small proportion of patients during the onset of hepatitis C and most patients with chronic HCV are not jaundiced. The development of jaundice, most often first noticed when the whites of the eyes go yellow, is a sign that the liver damage has increased very significantly and that you should seek urgent medical attention.

Portal hypertension   A condition called 'portal hypertension' can develop during cirrhosis. This happens when blood from the intestines can no longer flow through the liver because of scarring and pressure builds up within the blood vessels in the abdomen. Blood has to return to the heart, and any major obstruction leads to the development of bypass channels; so this increase in pressure causes blood from the gut to find an alternative route back to the heart.

The bypass channels usually form in the lining of the stomach and gullet (oesophagus). They are called 'varices' and are rather like the varicose veins that some people develop on their legs. Swollen varices can rupture and bleed. This bleeding (variceal haemorrhage) can be severe and cause the patient to vomit blood or pass bloody stools. Variceal bleeding is a feared complication of cirrhosis because it is sometimes fatal.

If you have cirrhosis and you vomit blood, you should call an ambulance immediately. In hospital the doctors will use a variety of drugs to reduce the pressure in the damaged blood vessels. They will also perform a special examination of the stomach (an endoscopy) with a fibre-optic telescope to see how serious the problem is. This is an uncomfortable procedure that is ordinarily carried out under light sedation.

In some cases bleeding from varices can be rather slow and the blood is not vomited up. As a result, the blood passes through the intestines where it is partially digested. It appears as black, smelly diarrhoea (melaena). If you notice that your motions go black, you should tell your doctor at once.

Encephalopathy   Because blood displaced in portal hypertension circumvents the liver, it tends to contain high levels of ammonia, amino-acids and other poisons. When these toxins get to the brain, they cause hepatic encephalopathy, which means 'liver-caused mental impairment'. The symptoms can range from subtle mental changes to profound confusion and coma.

In vulnerable patients encephalopathy can be brought on by a variety of relatively minor illnesses. For example, a trivial chest or urine infection can render someone with cirrhosis very confused. Constipation can sometimes be sufficient to precipitate an episode of encephalopathy, and patients should ensure that their bowels are opened at least once a day.

The treatment for encephalopathy is to clear the toxins from the bowel to stop them being absorbed. The medication usually prescribed is lactulose, a sweet-tasting laxative, which is helpful in cleaning the bowel. Many patients with cirrhosis take a small dose of lactulose every day to prevent constipation and reduce the risk of encephalopathy.

Ascites and oedema   Ascites is the swelling of the abdomen; oedema is the puffing up of the feet, legs or back. Both are due to fluid retention brought about by cirrhosis and portal hypertension.

These symptoms need to be treated with a low-salt diet, since salt encourages water retention in the body, and a restricted fluid intake. Most patients with ascites are able to drink a litre or so of fluid a day (just over two pints). A diuretic (water tablet) is often recommended to help the kidneys excrete more sodium and water.

At first you may find it difficult to adjust to these inconveniences, and it will probably take you a few weeks to become used to them. In particular, because of the limit imposed on the intake of fluids, it is likely that you will feel very thirsty while you adapt to the new regime. Sucking an ice cube helps to reduce this discomfort.

Asymptomatic Hepatitis

In some cases of chronic hepatitis patients do not realize that they are seriously ill until they reach end-stage liver disease. They have no symptoms and are said to be 'asymptomatic'. In this respect the virus is cunning, creating the illusion of good health in its victim while it bores away at the liver.

Larry had no noticeable effects of his chronic hepatitis until he nearly died of bleeding varices. Surgery was successfully completed and he was placed on a waiting list for a new liver:

'I retired from the military after twenty-three years in September 1993 and returned to university to complete my master's degree. Everything was just fine until 11 November of that year. A short time after eating dinner I began to feel ill. I was bloated despite having a light meal and I just couldn't get comfortable in any position. I went to bed and even then I was fidgety.

'My wife tucked me in for the night and headed out for her weekly evening with the girls. Shortly afterwards I became nauseous and the urge to throw up was over-whelming. I barely made it to the bathroom before what seemed like gallons upon gallons of blood came flowing out of me. There I stayed almost three hours, too weak to get up and call for help.

'When my wife arrived home she found me lying in the lavatory, unconscious and in shock. After being taken to hospital my prognosis was labelled poor and my wife was informed that it would be touch and go.

'I can recall waking up in intensive care, and standing

next to me were my wife, a priest and several doctors. I was being administered the last rites.

'I survived by the grace of God, but in December 1994 I began to bleed again. This time I was subjected to a six-hour surgical procedure that re-routed the arteries around my liver. They completed the operation successfully and I haven't had any more episodes of bleeding.

'I am now waiting for a transplant.'

Lifestyle Management

If you go on to end-stage liver disease, it is important that you adopt a sensible lifestyle. Four key areas to which you should pay strict attention are alcohol, diet, exercise and medication.

Alcohol
The advice here is straightforward: stop drinking immediately. Alcohol is metabolized by the liver and in large doses causes injury.

You should note that cirrhosis caused by hepatitis C progresses even more rapidly in patients who drink alcohol.

Diet
It is essential to eat the right kind of food. You will need to consult your doctor and probably enlist the help of a dietitian. For some patients, restrictions on salt intake will be necessary; other special diets will be recommended depending on particular symptoms. If you have ascites or oedema, you can reduce your sodium intake by avoiding such things as tinned soups and vegetables, crisps and cold meats. Fresh produce is preferred to prepared food, since the latter contains large amounts of salt used as preservative and flavouring.

Exercise

You must exercise regularly unless you are exhausted by even slight activity. Obviously, exercise is out of the question for those who are bedbound, but people in the early stages of decompensated cirrhosis may find that they get out of shape by doing nothing and suffer unnecessarily severe fatigue as a result. This kind of tiredness can be overcome.

You are not required to work out in a gym, although if you can it is a good idea. The best forms of exercise are swimming, jogging and walking. With all three, you can determine how much to do and how strenuously to do it. Remember: easy does it – but do it!

Medication

You should avoid all medication that is not essential. Drugs contain toxins which even a healthy liver finds hard to absorb, and some medications cannot be processed at all by people with advanced cirrhosis. Don't take any medication without discussing it with your doctor or pharmacist, even over-the-counter drugs.

It is essential that you avoid aspirin since this drug can increase the risk of bleeding. A surprisingly large number of cold and flu remedies contain aspirin. If you have a headache or other pain the safest painkiller is paracetamol, but you should be very careful not to take too much – a single tablet every six hours is usually a safe limit.

The Psychology of Suffering: Coping with End-Stage Liver Disease

A patient with active cirrhosis who enters end-stage liver disease faces a tough psychological adjustment. The illusion of longevity is shattered and the painful image of an abrupt end takes its place.

The dynamic of the disease changes from the threat of disabling symptoms to their reality. This depth of physical injury often undoes the sturdiest of constitutions. The need for care, love and support is felt more acutely than ever before. Those with systems of support in place find that they can approach the near-end, and the end if it comes to that, with some degree of equanimity. At both the practical and the emotional level they can put their affairs in order and confront with faith whatever happens.

Waiting to find out if you will get a transplant or if you will decline too far ever to receive one could destabilize you. Some people describe the wait as being on death row, although there is a very good chance of a reprieve.

Unlike a condemned prisoner, you have committed no capital crime. Your sense of injustice, rage and fear is likely to be enormous. A useful strategy is to prepare yourself mentally for this turbulent journey by acknowledging some of the emotions that will emerge.

A Sense of Injustice
It is horrific to recognize that you are dying and that you may not receive the new liver that can save your life, or may not survive a transplant even if a matching organ becomes available. It is desperately unfair that you are in this situation and that you are powerless over it. However, this does not mean there is nothing you can do with your feelings of injustice. Talk about them with your friends, family, self-help contacts or a counsellor.

Rage
Most people are furious that they are slowly dying. Life barely prepares us for life, let alone death. Your anger will intensify when you think about others who are getting the

very treatment that could save you. This kind of envy will chew into your guts and make your last days taste bitter. You will need an outlet for this pent-up frustration or you will make your final year a total misery.

Focusing on what has been good in your life is one way of dealing with rage and envy. Unlike people who die suddenly, say, from a stroke or car accident, you have a marvellous opportunity to seek redemption and reflect on what your life has meant to you and others. If you find enough room in your heart to be grateful for your life, but also to be willing to let it go, then it will be easier to accept your fate, whatever it turns out to be.

Fear
The most overwhelming emotion during the window period between the diagnosis of end-stage liver disease and the latest opportunity for a transplant is fear. Some are terrified that they will not receive a transplant before they become inoperable. Others cannot bear the suspense of the wait: 'Am I going to get a new liver?' 'Can I survive the operation?'

The reverse of fear is faith. Many turn to religion or therapy to find the inner strength to cope. Talking to others in the same position as you will help significantly. The therapeutic value of one pre-terminal patient consoling another is incalculable.

False Hope and Real Hope
A psychological pitfall awaits the unwary hoping for a transplant. All the talk with the surgeons and surviving patients will raise your expectations and can lead to living on false hope. You may assume that you will get the liver that you need and that the operation will be successful.

Neither is a foregone conclusion. You must recognize that you may not get a match and so pass through the window period during which you are fit enough to receive a transplanted organ. Alternatively, the right kind of liver may become available, but the surgery might kill or maim you instead. Do not be under any illusions about the risks and uncertainties involved.

On the other hand, it is a mistake to go to the other extreme and live in despair. Realistic hope is what you need.

Having a successful transplant is probably the only chance you have got of continuing your existence. If life is precious to you, you will be deeply grateful for this opportunity.

Most importantly, it provides grounds for limited optimism. There is a sporting chance that you will get a match for your liver and that you will come through the operation and recovery period successfully. During the dark days of decompensated cirrhosis, it can be a tremendous comfort to know that you are eligible for a transplant and that it could save your life.

Liver Failure and Transplants

The liver can be propped up for only so long by the short-term measures combating decompensated cirrhosis. Ultimately, the deterioration of this vital organ reaches a point of no return, and the liver fails entirely. It simply stops working and, unless a transplant is possible, the patient dies.

Unlike kidney or heart disease, there is no equivalent of a dialysis machine or heart pacemaker for damaged livers. At present someone with liver failure can be artificially supported for a few days, but this procedure is offered only if there is a possibility of a transplant.

Unfortunately, not everybody eligible for a liver transplant receives one because the correct match of organ is not always available. It is also a sad fact that many with end-stage liver disease are too ill to undergo such a major operation. And even if the operation is carried out, it is not always successful. The harsh reality is that half of those people with active cirrhosis are going to die from their complaint. If you enter end-stage liver disease, you may perish as a result of liver failure, complications, cancer, the shock of transplant surgery or the rejection of a new liver.

Nevertheless, the picture is not one of total gloom. A liver transplant was first performed on a human in 1963. Since then, surgical techniques have evolved rapidly and the survival rate has significantly increased. The chance of a successful transplant currently runs at over 80 per cent. Success in this instance means that the patient can return to, and fully enjoy, normal or near-normal life within about a year of the operation.

Many people with end-stage liver disease are eligible for a transplant. When they become aware of this life-saving possibility, their spirits lift as light appears at the end of the tunnel. To regain virtually full health after being in a pre-terminal condition is an amazing prospect.

The Specialist's Decision

It is up to a panel of doctors and health care workers to determine if you are a suitable candidate for a transplant. Your input and that of your family is taken into account, as well as the medical opinion of your hepatologist. In assessing your case, several factors are relevant. These include:

- *Need* You will only be considered for a transplant if you have end-stage liver disease or have sudden liver failure.
- *Age* Elderly patients are generally not offered a trans-

118

plant because their chances of survival are low. However, there is no upper age limit beyond which a transplant operation will not be performed, and people in their seventies who are otherwise fit have undergone successful transplants.

- *Physical condition* Your state of health apart from your liver problem will be taken into account. If you have other serious medical problems, like heart or lung disease, then the risks of transplantation are very high and you are unlikely to be placed on the waiting list.

- *Match* The only conditions that must hold between the donor and recipient are that they must be of approximately the same size and of compatible blood types. If you have a rare blood type, it will be difficult to find the right organ.

Other important concerns are availability and timing.

- *Availability* Healthy livers come from donors. Unfortunately there are not enough of them to go round. A liver is usually donated by someone who has consented prior to his or her death, or by next-of-kin where no prior consent is available. Livers for potential transplant are taken from those who have died in a number of ways, for example, through a fatal head injury due to a car accident.

- *Timing* There is a window period during which a patient's capacity to withstand major surgery is conducive to survival at the same time as liver disease necessitates a transplant. This is considered to be the last expected year of liver life. It is a dilemma that someone waiting for the right organ to be available may decline too far before one is ready for him. It is estimated that in America in 1992, 560 prospective recipients died while waiting for a liver.

Your Decision and Some of the Risks
If you are offered a place on a waiting list for a transplant, you should consider your position carefully. You must be aware of what the surgery involves, the consequences of having a transplant, and the difficulties of waiting for one.

With the actual operation come dangers attached to all forms of major surgery, such as dying under anaesthetic. In addition, there are the specific difficulties of removing the damaged liver and inserting the new one. The main problems are bleeding, poor function of the new liver, and bacterial infections.

Prior to the operation there is the possibility of developing a serious complication making you too weak to withstand major surgery. If this happens, you may not receive the liver that might otherwise have been yours.

It is an extremely difficult decision to make. In summary, the main risks are:

- You cannot predict whether the right organ will become available.
- You could die because of the shock of the surgery.
- You may reject the new liver.
- You will take a long time to recuperate and be on medication indefinitely.

Having a Transplant
You should count on spending several days in intensive care and then a few weeks in a general ward while recovering from the operation. In intensive care, all body functions, especially those of the liver, will be closely monitored. Once you are out of immediate danger, you will be transferred to the main ward.

For at least six weeks after transplantation, frequent tests are done to check on liver functions and to detect any signs of rejection. Should the grafted organ fail to function properly, it can be replaced if the circumstances permit.

David's experiences are typical of a transplant recipient:

'My need for a liver transplant became a reality in August 1994. I had asymptomatic hepatitis C which for a long time had been undiagnosed. I drank heavily in spite of my disease. Things became desperate when I got oesophageal varices.

'After six months of abstaining from alcohol, I was evaluated by my specialist and health care workers and accepted for a transplant. Then the waiting began. Although a part of me was hopeful because I was on a transplant waiting list, I also felt increasingly despondent as I watched myself wasting away and getting sicker and more forgetful every day.

'Out of the blue I was called at home and told to get immediately to the hospital. I was flustered and scared and reluctant to go.

'After I arrived at the hospital I was so busy with preparation that I honestly didn't have a chance to think about what was going on. Drugs, showers, enemas, shaving, answering a myriad of questions . . .

'I woke up in intensive care the next morning. My wife and my mother were there, waiting for me to regain consciousness.

'What I found unbearable were the respirator and my incredible thirst. I tried to take a gadget out of my mouth but my mother and the nurse stopped me. Later, I wrote a message to my mum and told her to go home and get some rest. While everyone had their backs turned I pulled that damnable thing out. Then I demanded some ice and threatened to go and get my own. I was in deadly earnest. What a relief those cool, wet cubes were!

'I was completely helpless and dependent on everyone for the slightest thing. With no stomach muscles, I couldn't even shift in bed by myself. My kidneys shut down for a while and the extreme discomfort was difficult for a few days. I guess swelling of the privates is common for men and women in this state.

'I was very fortunate. I was released from the hospital after only twelve days and am now taking care of myself quite well.

'Physically, I am stronger and better every day. I'm glad I had the transplant and I'm not about to waste valuable time worrying about the "what if" of rejection and the possibility of acute hepatitis C attack.

'I required constant care at home for two weeks while I recovered. My wife took a week off from work and my mother came to stay with us for another week after that. I would almost certainly be back in hospital without their help in maintaining my schedule: going to the chemist for batches of drugs, making my meals, and holding my hand.

'Now I believe in angels.'

The Rigours of Recovery

If you survive one year after your transplant, you are very likely to survive indefinitely. Many transplant patients have enjoyed full lives for ten or more years. If the operation goes well, you can expect not just to survive but to enjoy normal or near-normal life after one year. You could be walking within a week or two of the operation and should be able to participate in moderately vigorous exercise six to twelve months after leaving hospital. Sexual activity may be resumed when you wish, although the libido will be subdued for a while. The surgery is a shock to the system and the medication is strong.

Various drugs are used to facilitate acceptance of the new organ by the host body. Each kind has its own side-effects. A particular concern is that they tend to lower the patient's resistance to infection and to the development of tumours. Drugs from the cortisone family lead to fluid retention and puffiness around the face, the risk of worsening diabetes, if the patient is diabetic, and the possibility of depleting minerals in the bone marrow. Cyclosporin A can bring about high blood pressure and a growth of body hair. The dose of this drug has to be carefully regulated to avoid kidney damage.

You should note that anti-rejection drugs have to be taken for the rest of your life, although, as the new organ is accepted, the amounts of medication required are reduced.

Viral Hepatitis and the New Liver

Hepatitis C attacks the second liver and patients who survive a transplant invariably become reinfected with the virus. Treatment for recurrence of HCV infection rarely succeeds in such patients and the long term outcome is unclear. The vast majority will survive for the first five years without serious consequences, although there is concern that the virus may attack the new liver more aggressively than it attacked the old one. In a few transplantees the virus attacks the new liver furiously, and in some unfortunate patients the grafted liver fails within two years of the operation.

You should be comforted by the fact that there is a great deal of research going on to address the difficulties faced by transplant patients. Hepatologists hope that they may soon have a solution to the problem of recurrent HCV.

Conclusion

Entering end-stage liver disease can be like stepping into a dark lagoon. Everything is inky black and the only discernible direction is downwards into a terrifying unknown.

You must face this danger with all your courage. A thin ray of light is offered by the possibility of a transplant. This becomes a beam of hope, if you are eligible for surgery. It grows into solid ground for the chance of a new life, if you come through the operation.

Until recently, the notion of a successful transplant was only theoretical. Nowadays, it is an exciting reality. You may have the opportunity to recover from a condition that used to be fatal in every case.

9

Special Cases

Every patient with HCV can have his or her own particular problems. These vary depending upon whether the patient is a haemophiliac, a current or former drug user, a prisoner, a health care worker, a heavy drinker, a blood recipient, infected with other viruses too – or someone who falls into more than one of these groups.

The peculiarities attached to each set of circumstances range over the speed with which the disease develops and the suitability of treatment. For example, in the case of a heavy drinker the progression of the disease is accelerated, while for someone with HIV a liver transplant is out of the question.

Haemophiliacs

Haemophilia is a blood disease in which an essential clotting factor (usually factor VIII) is partially or wholly lacking. As a consequence, a haemophiliac can bleed for longer than normal. Although external wounds are not generally dangerous, internal bleeding into joints, muscles or soft tissues may be. Internal wounds can cause tremendous pain and result in disabilities. If they are untreated, they can be life-threatening.

Treatment for haemophilia consists of replacing the missing blood factor. This involves injections of concentrated clotting factors derived from donated blood, and because many thousands of different blood donors contribute to each batch of concentrate there is a high risk of infection from blood-borne diseases.

Before 1986 all concentrates could have been contaminated with HIV and HCV as the significance of these diseases was unknown at that time. Since 1986 people who have used intravenous drugs have been discouraged from giving blood, and although this policy was introduced to limit the transmission of the virus causing AIDS, a welcome benefit was a significant reduction in the number of donors infected with HCV.

Since 1991 all blood donors in the United Kingdom, the United States and most other countries have been screened for HCV and the risk of transmission through blood products is now extremely small. However, it is estimated that up to 90 per cent of British haemophiliacs who received clotting factors before this date were infected. Of the 9,000 haemophiliacs in Britain, there are 1,200 cases of HIV and 3,000 cases of HCV infection. Some have both viruses as well as other infections.

Haemophilia and HCV
Haemophiliacs with a single chronic infection follow the standard pattern of progress through the stages of the hepatitis cycle. The UK Haemophilia Centre Directors' Organization recommends drug treatment for all those with chronic infection who are not in end-stage liver disease.

The treatment of a patient with haemophilia is essentially the same as for an ordinary patient. However, for a haemophiliac the risks of undergoing a liver biopsy are much greater than normal, because of the danger of internal bleeding. This problem can be overcome by performing the biopsy through a vein in the neck (trans-jugular biopsy). A special needle is passed through a suitable blood vessel into the liver, where the biopsy is taken. If the liver bleeds, the blood goes back into the circulation and none is lost.

An alternative approach is to perform the biopsy through a small telescope passed, under local anaesthetic, directly into the abdomen. This allows the surgeon to see the liver during the biopsy, and if there is any bleeding the liver can be sealed using a heat probe. Although this approach sounds drastic, it is in fact almost painless.

Since a liver biopsy is far from straightforward in patients with haemophilia, many centres do not perform the procedure. If you are a haemophiliac with HCV, you should discuss the risks and benefits of a biopsy carefully with your specialist.

It is often the case that haemophiliacs are simply prescribed interferon regardless of the extent of the liver damage. The chances of a long-term response are the same as for non-haemophiliacs, namely 25 per cent.

A liver transplant will be considered for those whose cirrhosis is so advanced that they have a life expectancy of less than one year. A bonus for haemophiliacs having a transplant is that the new liver should produce enough clotting factors to preclude the further use of concentrate. In effect, they are cured of their blood condition.

Haemophilia, HIV and HCV

Those haemophiliac patients who have HIV and HCV infections are at grave risk from both viruses (see the section below on co-infected patients). Not only do co-infected haemophiliacs run the risk of all the problems associated with HIV, but they also have no hope of surgery as a last resort. Such a bleak prognosis makes stringent demands upon the mental resources of these patients.

Current Drug Users

Current drug users run the highest risk of infection and re-infection with HCV of all groups. Because of their tendency to share needles or other drug-using apparatus such as spoons or filters, addicts can easily inject themselves with the virus. It is estimated that over 70 per cent of drug users in the United Kingdom are infected with HCV, and similar rates have been reported from other countries around the world.

Specialists are often reluctant to treat using addicts with interferon because of the associated risks:

- Drug users often have a poor record of adhering to the discipline of interferon therapy. Since interferon is a potentially dangerous drug (suicidal depression and severe bone marrow suppression can occur), it is essential that patients taking interferon receive regular follow-up and medical supervision.
- Monitoring interferon therapy requires regular blood tests to be performed. Patients who have used or are still using drugs have often damaged their veins by injecting them with toxic drugs. This can make it very difficult to perform the requisite blood tests.
- There is concern that the use of needles for treatment with interferon may raise the chances of a relapse in those who have recently stopped taking drugs intravenously.
- There is a risk of re-infection with HCV even if interferon is successful in the first instance. If you live in an environment where many of your peers have HCV and you share their injecting equipment, it will not take long for you to catch the virus again, assuming you were able to clear it in the first place.

Although most doctors are reluctant to treat patients who are currently using drugs, many will treat addicts who abstain from intravenous drug-taking for six months or more, or who are committed to a programme of treatment with methadone.

A *Strategy for Current Drug Users*
If you are a using addict and you have chronic hepatitis, it is best to sort out your addiction problem first. Once you are clear of the dangers of a relapse, then get your liver disease treated. Narcotics Anonymous, a worldwide fellowship of recovering addicts, is a good starting point for those who want to learn how to live clean and sober (see 'Useful Addresses' at the end of this book).

For those who persist in injecting drugs, it is advisable to follow some simple rules in order to minimize the risk of infection or re-infection:

- Be careful to use clean needles, and *never* share them.
- Make sure your used needles are properly disposed of.
- Sterilize your injecting equipment (spoon, hypodermic, etc.).
- Keep your old needles and paraphernalia out of reach of curious children.
- *Never* borrow a spoon or other using equipment from someone else. It is known that HCV may be transmitted by routes other than intravenous injection, since some drug users who have never shared needles do become infected.

Former Intravenous Drug Users

A tragic fact of life for a large proportion of former intravenous drug users is that they have chronic hepatitis

C. It is often the case that a recovering addict has been out of the drug scene for many years when he or she discovers the past catching up with him or her. The patient begins to feel ill or has a routine check-up and with horror finds out that he or she has hepatitis C.

If you fall into this category, it is likely that the impact of this bad news will be shocking. You have worked extremely hard to detach yourself physically and psychologically from the compulsion to use drugs, only to learn that you injected yourself ages ago with something that might be fatal.

It takes a lot of courage to get back on your feet again. The only comfort is that someone who can kick the drug habit – and many cannot – has the internal resources to deal with chronic hepatitis. In time, your spirits will rise again and you will be able to face your new status.

The good news is that you fall into the 'healthiest' group apart from 'opportunistic' patients (see below). Assuming you drink no, or very little, alcohol and look after yourself physically and emotionally, you stand a reasonable chance of a moderately paced advance through the hepatitis cycle. Furthermore, if you undergo interferon or combination therapy, your lack of complications will be a positive factor in favour of a response.

William, who had been in recovery from active addiction for more than a decade, was disturbed when he found that he had a serious health problem stemming from his former way of life:

'I'd been clean and sober for over ten years when I found out that I'd got hepatitis C. I was devastated. I'd hoped that all the damage arising from my addiction had been sorted out many years previously.

'I went to get tested because many of my friends had done so and some of them were positive had also felt ill in an indiscernible way for a long time. I kept feeling tired for no obvious reason and often I got slight swellings in my throat. I tended to feel run down, even when I'd had a holiday.

'The symptoms I had were a nuisance that I tolerated for the most part. They were not really severe enough for me to think that there was anything especially wrong with me. I was shocked when the doctor said that I'd got hepatitis C and that I had extensive liver damage and would need treatment. I was frightened of injecting myself again after so many years. It was difficult for me to regard interferon as medication rather than a foul mood-altering substance.

'By attending self-help groups and talking to people in the same boat as myself, I was able to undergo this stern ordeal. I was relieved when I got used to the injections and I did not go back to drugs.'

Prisoners

If you are in prison, there is a grave danger of acquiring hepatitis C. A small, voluntary study of sixteen prisoners found that six of them had HCV infection, while they were negative for HIV, syphilis and hepatitis B. The sample did not include drug addicts.

It is imperative that prison inmates follow the basic anti-infection guidelines. In particular:

- *Do not* share the razors, toothbrushes or nail files of other prisoners;
- *Do not* get tattooed or body-pierced or have an earring put in;
- *Never* share drug equipment.

If you are in prison and are already infected, not only must you follow these guidelines, but you must realize you are unlikely to be treated. Because you are in such a closed and infectious environment, your specialist, if you have access to one, will recommend that you wait until after you are released.

Those Infected at Work

Doctors, nurses, dentists and other health care workers are at risk of infection by the very nature of their work. Those who are in contact with hepatitis patients on a regular basis may catch the virus through two routes:

- *percutaneous exposure*, where the skin is cut or pene- trated by a needle or other sharp object, for example a scalpel blade, bone fragment or tooth, which is con- taminated by blood;
- *mucocutaneous exposure*, where the eye or eyes, the inside of the mouth, or an area of non-intact skin is contaminated by blood.

It is current practice to treat health care workers who have active liver disease with interferon or combination therapy as soon as possible, even if they have no liver damage. The reason for this is to prevent their infecting others in the course of pursuing their duties.

Opportunistic Patients

This class includes all those who do not know how they have acquired the virus. They cannot have been infected by blood, intravenous drug use or sexual transmission, and have not worked with hepatitis patients. It is a medical mystery how such people become infected.

In Australia it is believed that in up to 20 per cent of

hepatitis C cases no obvious contact with the virus can be identified. This raises many issues about the manner of HCV transmission, which researchers are currently investigating.

The problem for this group is that no one within it suspects prior to their diagnosis that they have viral hepatitis. They only find out about their infection when they have a general check-up or are tested for some other reason and liver function abnormalities are revealed. For example, a number of former blood donors who fall outside all the obvious risk categories have been diagnosed with hepatitis C since screening procedures have been introduced.

It appears that many undiagnosed patients are going about their daily lives with no inkling that they have a dangerous infection – with the obvious consequent hazard that they are putting at risk anyone who comes into contact with their blood.

Blood Recipients

Blood transfusion has been one of the main risk factors for transmission of HCV. Unfortunately, the hepatitis C virus was only identified in 1989 and before then it was impossible to test blood for the presence of the virus – no one knew what to look for! Now that blood products are screened for infections, this route of transmission will close.

Heavy Drinkers

Anyone diagnosed with hepatitis C who drinks heavily is committing suicide. This is pouring paraffin on to a fire. When a drinker's liver becomes cirrhotic, he or she can expect to live only five years or so.

Most specialists will not treat heavy drinkers who have HCV with interferon or combination therapy unless and until they stop abusing themselves. Alcoholic liver disease is as rampant as viral hepatitis, but is clearly preventable if the patient can stop drinking.

Heavy drinkers are unlikely to be recommended for liver transplant unless they follow a programme of strict abstinence. The argument is that those drinkers who have received new livers and have survived long enough to get out and about then go back to alcohol as soon as they can. Their new livers malfunction and the precious organs go to waste.

If you are an HCV patient and a compulsive drinker, you had best stop drinking immediately. Go to Alcoholics Anonymous to get help with your problem (for details see 'Useful Addresses' at the end of this book). If you are able to control your drinking, then reduce your intake to what is considered a harmless level, that is, twenty one units a week for a man, fourteen units a week for a woman (a unit is half a pint of beer, a small glass of wine, or a bar measure of spirits). Spread your allowance out: don't abstain for six days and then binge out on Saturday!

Co-infected Patients

There are many varieties of viral co-infection. This section covers some of the main ones with which distinct problems are associated.

HIV and HCV

Dual infection with the virus that leads to AIDS, the HIV virus, and hepatitis C is rare. In the past patients with both viral infections have been most concerned about HIV, since this virus kills people more quickly than hepatitis C. It is a sad fact that for many people with dual infections death from HIV and its complications has occurred so quickly that the problems of HCV have not had time to develop. This gloomy picture has recently begun to change. A large number of new drugs that inhibit the replication of the HIV virus, antiretrovirals, have been developed, and these have dramatically changed the prognosis for patients with this infection. Many patients with quite advanced HIV infection are treated successfully and their HIV infection goes into remission.

The dramatic improvement in life expectancy for patients with HIV has led to an increasing awareness of the possible effects of HCV in such patients. It is likely that many with dual infections will survive for long enough for HCV to cause significant liver problems. This possibility has led some clinicians to treat patients with HIV and HCV with drugs that are active against HCV, chiefly ribavirin and interferon. Although only a few patients have been treated in this way, it appears that the combination of antiretrovirals, which suppress the HIV infection, and interferon plus ribavirin can cure some patients of their HCV infection. Clearly, these treatment regimes are very demanding and require patients to take very large numbers of tablets and injections. You should think very carefully about the difficulties of managing all these different medicines before embarking on this therapy.

HBV, HCV and HDV
Some patients have a variety of chronic viral infections. A particularly troublesome combination is hepatitis B, C and D. HBV and HCV are serious enough on their own; when accompanied by HDV or delta hepatitis, the progression of the disease may be extremely rapid.

People with this kind of co-infection usually require

early treatment to stem the viral torrent. Unfortunately the presence of multiple viruses may reduce the chances of a successful response to interferon.

HCV and HGV
An increasing number of people are being found to have these two infections. HGV has only recently been identified. It is thought that one-fifth of those infected with HCV also carry HGV.

It is not yet known how dual infection of this kind affects interferon therapy, but current data suggest that co-infection with HGV is not a significant problem and neither speeds up the rate of liver damage nor reduces the chance of responding to interferon.

Conclusion

Each category of HCV patient has its own problems. It is essential that you find out what the particular conditions are that relate to your particular group, and find out all you can about your state of health. Your specialist can help you.

There are no definitive formulae concerning HCV, as medical records of the virus are so far inconclusive. This is both a burden and a joy. It is a burden because you must do the footwork – no one can say precisely either how your infection will progress or what particular treatment is the best for you. It is a joy because you can grow through this experience of breaking new ground.

10

Personal Stories

The personal accounts collected in this chapter show how chronic hepatitis C affects certain people and how they live with it. These individuals have collectively experienced a wide range of symptoms. Some are single and young; others are married, or middle-aged. Each has found a unique way of dealing with long-term illness, and although no one reader's experience will exactly match any of these examples, there is much to be learned from them.

What these people have in common is that they have all asked for help in one way or another, and are all courageously confronting a health problem that threatens to shorten their lives. They offer hope, without giving false hope.

Jim's Story

Jim lives in Alaska, USA, and caught hepatitis C as a result of a blood transfusion. He had been involved in a car accident. Although his quality of life is beginning to sag and he worries about the future, he is able to live his life to the full and enjoy the presence of his family. He has tried western herbal remedies as a treatment for HCV:

'When I was a paper boy, I used to do the round on a motorbike. One morning I got hit broadside by a Cadillac and was seriously injured. Since then, I have had a bunch of surgery. I can't recall the exact number of operations, but it was during one of them that I picked up hepatitis C.

'I was constantly told that there was little danger of infecting others and that there was no fail-safe treatment available. Most of the time I felt OK and forgot about it. Now my disease has become aggressive and will not be ignored.

'I'm not dead yet. When I look in the mirror something alive still looks back at me. So I'm trying to cram stuff into my new time frame: kids, career, hopes and dreams. All these things need attending to. And everything is moving at a new speed. Five and ten year plans look different. I call it "accelerated life".

'Just this moment I feel happy. My eight-year-old son is at the kitchen table, making me a multi-coloured necklace of Indian corn. A gentle rain is falling from a grey wash of Alaskan sky. The cat is purring at the window and my mug of milk thistle tea is hot . . . I think I'll put some of them necklaces in the café store where I work.'

James's Story

James, 36, from Somerset, England, is a counsellor in the management of chronic illness. He is a former intravenous drug user, who caught hepatitis C in his early twenties. Three years ago, James was bewildered by his symptoms and his local health services' ignorance of his condition. Although he has mild disease in terms of liver damage, he has had to adapt to certain physical and psychological limitations imposed upon him by hepatitis C. Through his work and personal experience James has developed a set of

general guidelines on how to take responsibility for himself
and his chronic condition:

'Shall I tell you about the many visits to the doctors over
the years with mystery symptoms and the tests for
everything from irritable bowel syndrome to anaemia
and diabetes that followed?

'Or the doctor who thought that I simply needed "to
get with it a bit more"?

'Or the General Practitioner (GP) I saw after testing
positive who informed me she didn't really know what I
expected her to do about it?

'Or the long, anxious twelve months waiting for a
biopsy, swinging between being convinced I had liver
cancer to feeling that, well, maybe I do need "to get with
it a bit more"?

'This all happened three years ago and I am pleased to
say that where I am in Bath things are a bit better.

'I am fortunate in that I still have time on my side. I
have mild disease and limited liver damage and I do not
want to take interferon yet. As such I am one of those
who sees the specialist once a year. I see the GP very
occasionally, when I get a bit paranoid and have my liver
function tests carried out.

'That leaves 364 days and nights when I don't have
the support of a professional hepatologist. It's just me
and my virus. For the foreseeable future, I am stuck with
it.

'This gives me a simple choice. I can be a victim of the
virus – angry, resentful, blaming the health service for not
coming up with a fail-safe cure or myself for getting it in
the first place. Or I can become proactive – take on the
responsibility for managing the illness on a daily basis and
make the necessary decisions and take the necessary
actions to keep myself as healthy and happy as possible.

'To be proactive, I need up-to-date and reliable information, emotional support and a network of self-help. In other words, I need a partnership with other people like me, my family and health care professionals.

'There are three areas for which I take responsibility.

1) *My Illness*: I take medication as and when directed. I have made appropriate lifestyle changes, kept hospital and GP appointments, stayed informed about treatment developments.
2) *Normal Activities*: I maintain my personal appearance and hygiene, and I work, if only part time. I also keep up a social life.
3) *Emotional Changes:* I manage the emotional changes brought about by my illness, which include anger, uncertainty about the future, depression and shifts of power in my friendships and relationships.

'By doing all these things, I have accepted the limits placed upon me by hepatitis C and learned to flourish within them.'

Dave's Story

Dave is from Birmingham, Alabama, USA. He led a drunken lifestyle for many years and does not know how he caught hepatitis, although it may have been sexually transmitted as he has a multiple infection. He underwent interferon therapy and was a non-responder. He also tried complementary medicine, but with similarly disappointing results. Nevertheless, he lives in the hope of a cure being discovered:

'In 1982 I was coming to the end of my drinking period. I had been living in Birmingham with my brother, where we owned a bar. Most of my days and nights were spent doing quality control checks on the draught beer. Even though I was 30 years old, the only recourse I had for cleaning up my act was to move in with my parents for a while.

'My folks insisted that I see a doctor and I had various medical tests. He said that I had alcoholic hepatitis and suggested that I stop drinking, which I did.

'Six months later my liver function tests were still abnormal and I was referred to a hepatologist. I was given a biopsy, which showed that I had chronic persistent hepatitis, and was found to be positive for hepatitis B.

'I had no idea when I got the disease. It could have been a year or ten years prior to the test. There was no way of telling.

'Since I didn't feel too bad, I went on my merry way. I was a pretty active person: I jogged 15 miles a week and went mountaineering every chance I got. I had six-monthly check-ups. My only symptom was occasionally suffering fatigue. It was expected that the disease would disappear of its own accord eventually. That was that, or so I thought.

'It wasn't, though. The disease didn't clear itself and I began to feel worse. In 1990 I was tested for hepatitis C and was found to be positive.

'The medically accepted treatment was interferon alpha, which I underwent. It was very expensive and I had to pay for it myself as I was uninsured. For six months I took three million units three times a week, to which I didn't respond. My LFTs were still abnormal. I was prescribed a higher dose, five million units three times a week. A slight improvement occurred, but not a significant one. So I discontinued the treatment.

'My quality of life has deteriorated over the last several years. My overall level of fatigue has increased dramatically and I have abdominal and joint pains, which are severe at times. I've seen acupuncturists, Chinese herbalists and homeopaths with varying degrees of success. None of these has produced any sustained improvement in my LFTs or my symptoms. My latest biopsy indicated cirrhosis, although I haven't been placed on a transplant list yet.

'All I can do is live as carefully as I can, eat well, and get as much sleep as I need. Like most people with hepatitis C, I'm hoping for that magic bullet to come along that will wipe out all these viruses.'

Sara's Story

Sara from the US caught the virus through intravenous drug use. She has had it for many years and has experienced some painful symptoms. Her way of coping is to attend local support groups:

'As close as I can tell I injected HCV into my veins in 1972 or 1973. For about one and a half years I partied hard and indulged in many forms of high-risk behaviour with no eye on the future. I was in my mid-twenties and thought myself invincible.

'In 1973 I became sick and was diagnosed as having non-A non-B hepatitis. I lost about fifteen pounds, which I could not afford to, and I was always exhausted.

'I was married to my second husband at the time, who was an alcoholic. I drank right along with him, sick as I was. I didn't eat much and I was smoking cigarettes and quaffing cheap wine.

'I left him in January 1974 and spent the next few years being abstemious. I occasionally smoked pot, but did no more hitting up or drinking. In 1979 I gave up illegal drugs, although I continued to smoke and drink coffee.

'I married my third husband in 1980. I felt healthy and energized and had no real trouble apart from two bouts of kidney stones, one in 1985 and the other in 1988. I was fine! I could eat anything.

'In 1991 I started getting what I thought was severe heartburn. I couldn't figure it out. The pain was concentrated on my right side under my rib cage and it would shoot up my side all the way into my throat. I thought I was on fire inside. My throat was permanently a little bit sore. I gave up smoking and that helped some. The pain would lie dormant for a period of time and then it would return full force.

'I was also suffering from itching that I couldn't put a cause to. The tops of my feet and my ankles itched so much at times that I couldn't wait to get home and tear off my socks. And my head, sides and stomach would itch as well.

'By the end of 1993 I was divorced from my third husband. Early in the following year I changed physicians, too. I told my new doctor about the pain in my gut and he did various tests. In February 1994 I was told that I was positive for hepatitis C. At first, I tried to laugh it off. I didn't take it seriously because I didn't know anything about it.

'I learned things about HCV and became worried since I had had active hepatitis for so long and because of my relentless symptoms. I became angry that I had this problem and that it could kill me.

'I began attending support group meetings in March 1995, which I have found very helpful. I also undergo regular monitoring to keep a check on my LFTs.

'The worst thing about this disease for me is the idea that I am poisoned and poisonous. I cannot donate blood or organs and I must be careful about not passing on the infection.'

Anthony's Story

Anthony is a family man, working in London, who has vacillated about receiving interferon therapy. He has tried complementary remedies, and finally took the new pegylated interferon as part of a trial. To help himself live with his chronic condition, he talks regularly to other hepatitis patients on the telephone:

'In 1989 I went for a medical check-up because my business partner had died suddenly of cancer and I was anxious in case there was something wrong with me. The doctor found there was a slight abnormality in my liver function. Initially, he attributed it to the nature of my recent past – I had been a heavy drinker and drug user. Then, he phoned me a few weeks later and said he had discussed my case with a colleague and that he advised my going to King's College Hospital for further blood tests.

'The specialist took some of my blood and asked me to return in a few weeks. When I saw him again I was told in front of a crowd of medical students that I had chronic hepatitis C and that it was a very serious illness with three possible outcomes: cirrhosis, cancer or clearing the virus. He said I'd got a fifteen- to twenty-year period free of complications.

'I felt angry at the insensitive way I had been told, and I was alarmed that I'd got an illness with potentially dangerous consequences. I was also scared of the treatment that he talked about which was interferon by injection.

'It wasn't a surprise there was something wrong with me because I'd often felt tired and generally run down. I'd been prepared to put that down to my age – over 40 – and my busy life. I didn't have any screaming symptoms, just a vague feeling of being unwell.

'I was told that the infection was only rarely sexually

transmitted, but that as a precaution my wife should be tested. She was HCV negative. We were trying to have a child at the time so we didn't employ safe sex.

'These days I'm careful if I get a cut. I wash it and bandage it immediately. I'm particularly vigilant about my blood or saliva when I'm with the young boy we've had. I don't let him or my wife use my toothbrush or handle my razor.

'Once I got over my initial fear of having hepatitis C, I tended to blank the whole issue. I just didn't want to face it. As time has gone on, my awareness of my illness has built up. I'm unhappy to have this problem, but I'm relieved that I'm in better health than many others with HCV.

'I sometimes feel stigmatized. "HCV" sounds like "HIV" or at least falls into a similar category so far as public awareness is concerned. When I discuss my disease with people who don't know anything about it, they seem to think I've got AIDS. I suffer from other people's ignorance and prejudice.

'I don't drink alcohol, I don't smoke, I don't drink coffee very much. I'm careful about my diet – I don't often eat cheese or fatty foods. The stuff that gets to me is greasy cuisine like sausages and fried eggs. If I eat these things, I feel like I've got a hangover. So I avoid them.

'Since I've been monitored, my LFTs have ranged between 70 and 100. I had my first liver biopsy four or five years ago, which showed that I had chronic active hepatitis C. There was no scarring, but there was evidence of the virus munching away at the healthy cells.

'The clinic offered me interferon and I wasn't very keen on trying it. I put off making a positive decision. Then the doctor affirmed that the treatment had better results for those early in the hepatitis cycle and I was tempted again. I liked the idea of a long-term benefit, that is, clearing the virus in exchange for a short-term discomfort – taking the medication. I decided to try it, but never got round to it. I dillied and dallied and then put it back on hold.

'The whole palaver of being on interferon spooked me: injections, feeling ill, the side-effects, the fact that it might not work. Also, because I have my own business and have a young family, I didn't think that I could find the time to be on it. So, I didn't go on it when it was first recommended, hoping that something better would come along.

'For a year and a half I was on Chinese herbs. I saw a man who examined my tongue and asked me about my liver problem. He prescribed me some little black pellets and a brew of herbs, which I drank. It's hard to say if it did any good. It certainly did no harm. My LFTs remained in the same range they had been since I'd attended the liver unit.

'The most useful thing I do is belong to a telephone network of fellow hepatitis sufferers. I phone some of them up from time to time and often someone calls me. We talk about the latest information on hepatitis and how we have been getting on with our diseases – what they've been doing, what I've been doing about it.

'It's helpful to hear from people who are at the same stage of the viral problem as myself and to learn about people who are further down the slope. I don't know how it works, but I get a lot from sharing my feelings about hepatitis with other hepatitis sufferers. We can identify with each other and then I don't feel alone with it any more.

'A year ago, I had my second biopsy, which showed progressive liver fibrosis. My ALT and AST fluctuated above 120, whereas previously they had been well under 100. I was getting worse. The specialist at King's College Hospital offered me a place on a trial of pegylated interferon, which involved one rather than three injections a week. I took up the opportunity and am nine months into a year of treatment and was PCR negative at three and six months with normal LFTs. I am over the moon with my response, although I feel depressed and out of touch with my feelings because of the drugs. Initially, I was disturbed by taking the injection, but was pleased it was only once a week.

'The uncertainty of the future sometimes affects me. I'm scared that I'm going to relapse when I stop the interferon. How will I feel if the virus comes back and I get worse symptoms than before?

'I deal with the uncertainty by staying in the day. I'm OK just for today just as I am. I can enjoy my life in my current state of health and I'm keeping watch over myself. The rest is up to fate.'

Ricky's Story

It is not known how Ricky, who was born in Hertfordshire, England, acquired hepatitis C; he falls into three risk categories. He was terrified when he found out that he had cirrhosis and that his life would be cut short unless the virus was cleared. He is lucky in that he responded to conventional therapy and was still clear of the virus after the treatment ended:

'I don't know how I was infected as there are at least three ways that it might have occurred. When I was young I attended various boarding schools where it was a standard practice to inoculate children with the same needle. If child A had an infection, then all the children inoculated after him were at risk. So I could have caught it this way, especially as my mother remembers me being jaundiced when I was ten or eleven years old.

'In my late adolescence and early adulthood I was an

147

intravenous drug user. I do not recall sharing needles, as I found it hard enough to inject myself even with a fresh one. But this is certainly a well-known route of infection.

'Thirdly, I caught hepatitis B from a friend of mine who was sexually promiscuous. I may have had hepatitis C transmitted to me by performing penetrative sex.

'In 1984, I stopped using, one day at a time, and began to live in a more fruitful manner. Slowly I reinvented myself after my period of wantonness and drug abuse and began to take a genuine pleasure in my existence. I became happy for perhaps the first time in my life.

'When I got to my late thirties, I began to feel dreadfully ill for no apparent reason. I felt sick, exhausted, and sweated a lot both at night and during the day. I also had livid blemishes on my back and chest. My partner kept complaining about how irritable and slothful I was. If I tried to do any housework, I soon felt knackered. When we went on holiday, I tended to sleep the whole time.

'There always seemed to be a way of explaining my decline without considering serious illness. I had two occupations. I was a research student in philosophy at London University and I had a role in a family-owned business, managing property. My overworking was the reason why I felt ill, or so my partner and I deluded ourselves.

'In 1989 I was told that my liver was inflamed when I had blood tests during a general check-up. It was suggested that I have further tests. Because I wasn't in any immediate danger, I procrastinated.

'Some years later I was tested for HCV and my doctor misinformed me as to the result. When after a gap of two years I found out that I was positive, I complained bitterly about being misled. Eventually, I was referred to a specialist who gave me a biopsy. I was stunned when I was told that I had active cirrhosis and that I had only a

50 per cent chance of living for more than five years. I felt that I had been condemned to death. I was terribly upset because I thought that my life was over before it had really begun. I had spent many years recovering from addiction and now that my life was going well, it was all being snatched away from me.

'Once I got over the initial shock, I made enquiries about self-help groups and became part of a chain of telephone interlocutors who tell each other how they are getting on with their hepatitis C. I derived enormous hope and inspiration from these two sources of support.

'The clinic that I attended offered me treatment on the basis that I was seriously ill, but not so ill that I could not benefit. I took interferon alone for six months and my LFTs became normal. The virus did not clear and I was prescribed ribavirin in combination with interferon. I was frightened of taking this untested drug because the doctor warned me that they did not know how or if it worked. There was a danger of unknown side-effects. I tried the new therapy and to my delight I responded during the final half year of treatment. To my further surprise and pleasure, I was still in remission six months after I stopped the drugs. When I found out I burst into tears because I was so moved by the thought of actually clearing the virus.

'Becoming free of active liver disease after all I have been through is now a fantastic possibility. I have stayed clear of the virus for over two and a half years, and there is a very good chance that I will remain free of it indefinitely. I'm absolutely thrilled by this.'

Cheri's Story

Cheri who lives in Florida in the US, was successful in the competitive world of finance before being struck down by hepatic symptoms. Initially, they were attributed to a psychological disorder, even though she believed otherwise. Her disease caused her extreme distress and worry. It threatened not only her job but also her family life, illustrating that chronic disease has devastating consequences far beyond the discomfort of the patient. She found long sought-for support through the Internet:

'Before getting ill I had always been full of boundless energy. I worked in the mortgage banking industry for twenty-odd years and sang with bands at clubs and parties in the evenings. I became a specialist in my field and continued my education in banking. I gave and attended seminars, trained employees and finally made it up the corporate ladder to Vice President of Operations.

'Some time in early 1993 I began to have what seemed like repeated attacks of flu. I caught every cold or sniffle that came within miles of me. These attacks became worse and lasted for longer and longer periods of time.

'Instead of missing one day of work, I was starting to miss two, three and even four because I was so fatigued. My bones, joints and muscles hurt so much that I couldn't even get out of bed. It was exasperating to wonder not only what was wrong with me, but also whether or not I'd be able to keep my job in the business world.

'For a long while I had no diagnosis to fit my symptoms. The doctor thought that I was depressed and needed psychiatric help. Quite a few times I was told that what I was experiencing was in my mind and not my body. I was asked repeatedly why I wanted to be sick. It was so difficult to convince anybody that I didn't *want* to be ill, but that I *was* ill.

'My symptoms became alarming. I started to suffer from bouts of short-term memory loss. When I stood up from my desk after hanging up the phone, I couldn't remember why I had got up. On other occasions I would be on my way to the fax machine or the supply room and forget where I was going. I would continue out of the door and seek refuge in the lavatory trying to figure out what was wrong with me.

'Sometimes I would be driving at 70 miles an hour to or from work on the motorway and drift off somewhere, unable to concentrate or keep my mind on what I was doing. Also, I couldn't remember lyrics to songs I'd sung hundreds of times.

'When I was diagnosed as having hepatitis C in October 1994 I was relieved. Relieved that there was something medically wrong with me. Relieved that there was a treatment for it. But I was not happy with the way that others responded to my infection. At first, my husband and children were frightened of me because they were worried they might catch the virus. All but two sets of friends turned away for the same sort of reason.

'I was offered the chance of interferon therapy and was attracted by the possibility of remission. After discussing the difficulties of treatment with my family, I began the injections at the end of November 1994. It was horrible. I felt isolated in my home and very ill from the side-effects of the interferon. I had my pets and I had myself, but my husband was at work and my children at school. I spent many of those days huddled in a foetus position in my bed.

'No one else close to me understood what I was going through. My husband didn't even want to face it, much less talk about it. He gave me my injections and then went back into denial. I was in a very depressed state of mind: my marriage was getting rocky and I felt so alone. We both learned how serious an illness chronic active hepatitis really is.

'After what seemed like an eternity the treatment

came to an end with no lasting benefits. Yet my marriage weathered those stormy times. In the long run the difficulties have strengthened our relationship by questioning our loyalty to each other.

'Chronic hepatitis C is a very difficult disease to live with for all concerned. Many times I see and believe that the strain imposed by the disease in some way is easier on me than it is on my husband, son, daughter and other relations.

'A good thing is that my in-laws purchased a computer for us in November 1995. I subscribed to the Internet and the first keywords I typed were Hepatitis C. I followed the links and found a number of helpful sites. I wrote to two of the people, one female and one male. At last I had found others who were going through the same things that I was. I thank God that He led me there.'

Ed's Story

Ed, 38, from north Hampshire, England, is a director of a major property company. He caught hepatitis C while using drugs in France and began to notice symptoms in his early thirties, after he entered recovery from addiction. He has a young family and underwent mono- and dual therapy, achieving a long-term response. Although the drugs affected his thryroid gland, he is delighted to be clear of the virus many months after completing treatment:

'I caught hepatitis C sharing needles with someone in the Jardin des Anglais in Cannes. Generally, I was scrupulous about who I shared with, but I went for it in the South of France.

'When I stopped using, I was aware of having something wrong with my liver. It was swollen. I felt I'd got a football bladder under my right ribs, which someone was slowly pumping up. I was tired as well.

'I attended a liver unit and was diagnosed with hepatitis C. For several years, my ALT fluctuated mostly between 60 and 100, though it went up to 300 at one point. I had three biopsies in two years. The third showed progressive scarring.

'I was recommended interferon treatment by Dr Murray-Lyons at the Chelsea and Westminster Hospital, and because I wanted to do something about my disease, I started. I was on five mega-units three times a week and didn't have too rough a time, apart from the first few weeks. My ALT reduced to the lower 50s by the end of six months, but I didn't clear the virus.

'I was a bit negative . . . disappointed, but I'd been promised combination therapy if the interferon on its own didn't work. The doctor put me on 1200 mg – six capsules – a day of ribavirin on top of the interferon.

'To start off with, the only extra side-effect was a lot of itching, especially in my scalp. I got a lot of dandruff.

'Except for the last three months of treatment, I kept working full time. Ten until six at the office in London and two hours commuting each day on my motor bike.

'The cumulative effect of a year of combination treatment after six months of interferon took its toll. I lost weight, about 30–35 lb at one stage, and my hair dropped out in clumps. My energy level significantly reduced. From December 1997 to February 1998 – the last three months of my treatment – I worked only five hours a day, starting at ten and finishing at three. I stopped commuting on my motor bike and drove a car instead.

'My ability to perform socially and with my family diminished. I was getting tired much earlier than usual and going to bed earlier. I'm a naturally up person, but during treatment I was flat, withdrawn, and much snappier with my children – I've got five-year-old twins and a stepdaughter.

'I didn't go out much and played with the children much less, but I was given lots of support by my wife and friends and work colleagues. I had a lot of understanding at my job. They knew about my hepatitis C and my treatment, and didn't mind my working only part time.

'When I finished treatment, the itchy scalp and flaky skin got better. My hair thickened up. I also put on weight and became more energetic. I was back to normal in a couple of weeks.

'My hepatitis symptoms had gone. The sensation of having a football jammed under my ribs lifted.

'My only problem was thyroidism. For the last months of treatment my blood test results for thyroxine production were haywire. I ended up having a deficiency and needed to take 100 mcg of thyroxine a day. The dose has been reduced several times and I am now on 25 mcg a day. My readings are still slightly haywire ten months after treatment. The doctor is hopeful that he can wean me off it.

'I went PCR-negative soon after I began the dual therapy. It was a great feeling, to fight back and get the virus on the run. I didn't want to come off it, irrespective of any side-effects, until there was a good chance of a sustained response. I finished treatment about ten months ago and had normal LFTs with PCR-negative nine months later.

'It's been a success for me and I feel better than I have done for years. People, in particular those I haven't seen for a while, say I'm back to my old self.'

Useful Addresses

UNITED KINGDOM

Information on Hepatitis C

British Liver Trust (BLT)
Central House
Central Avenue
Ransomes Europark
Ipswich IP3 9QG
Helpline tel. 01473 276328
Freephone 0808 800 1000
Website http://www.britishlivertrust.org.uk
Email info@britishlivertrust.org.uk

The BLT produces a wide variety of pamphlets on many issues relating to liver disease as well as a regular publication, C *Positive*, which is a supplement of *Liver Focus*, their newsletter. They also keep an up-to-date list of local support groups.

Information on Liver Cancer

British Association of Cancer United Patients
3 Bath Place
Rivington Street
London EC2A 3JR
Helpline tel. 0171 608 1661

CancerLink
17 Britannia Street
London WC1X 9JN
Tel. 0171 833 2451

Self-Help Groups and Specialized Information

Chronic Disease Self-Management Courses
c/o Jim Phillips
67 Southdown Road
Bath BA2 1HL
Tel. 01225 353182
Email JimPhillips@cableinet.co.uk

Haemophiliacs
The Haemophilia Society
Chesterfield House
385 Euston Road
London NW1 3AU
Tel. 0171 380 0600
Fax. 0171 387 8220
Website http://www.haemophilia.org.uk
Email lucy@haemophilia.org.uk
Karin@haemophilia.org.uk

Former or Current Drug Users
Hep C Support Group
Box M006
Mainliners
205 Stockwell Road
London SW9 9SL
Tel. 0171 738 4656

Recovery from Addiction
Narcotics Anonymous
UK Service Office
202 City Road
London EC1V 2PH
Helpline tel. 0171 730 0009

Recovery from Alcoholism
Alcoholics Anonymous
Jacob House
3 Cynthia Street
London N1 9JE
Helpline Tel. 0171 833 0022

Testing and Storage of Semen
Diagnostic Andrology Centre
Bourn Hall Clinic
Bourn
Cambridge CB3 7TR
Tel. 01954 719111

Useful Addresses

Hospitals Offering Treatment for Hepatitis (London only)

The following hospitals have a particular interest in treating patients with viral hepatitis. Many other hospitals in London also provide treatment.

Charing Cross Hospital
Fulham Palace Road
London W6
Tel. 0181 383 0000

Chelsea and Westminster Hospital
369 Fulham Road
London SW10 9NH
Tel. 0181 746 8000

Kings College Hospital
Denmark Hill
London SE5 9RS
Tel. 0171 737 4000

Royal Free Hospital
Pond Street
London NW3 2QG
Tel. 0171 830 2823

St Bartholomew's Hospital
57 West Smithfield
London EC1
Tel. 0171 601 8888

St George's Hospital
Blackshaw Road
London SW17 OQT
Tel. 0181 672 1255

St Mary's Hospital
Praed Street
London W2 1PG
Tel. 0171 886 6666

Carers

Carers National Association
20-25 Glasshouse Yard
London EC1 4JS
Tel. 0171 490 8818
Fax. 0171 490 8824
CarersLine 0345 573 369 (office hours)

Complementary Treatment Centres (London only)

The Hale Clinic
7 Park Crescent
London W1N 3HE
Tel. 0171 631 0156

The Society for Complementary Medicine
31 Weymouth Street
London W1N 3FJ
Tel. 0171 436 0821

The Gateway Clinic
South Western Hospital
Landor Road
London SW9 9NU
Tel. 0171 346 5400

Professional Organizations for Complementary Treatments

British School of Reflexology
The Holistic Healing Centre
92 Sheering Road
Old Harlow
Essex CM17 0JW
Tel. 01279 429060

Institute for Complementary Medicine
21 Portland Place
London W1N 3AF
Tel. 0171 237 5165

National Institute of Medical Herbalists
56 Longbrook Street
Exeter
Devon EX4 6AH
Tel. 01392 426022

Register of the Society of Homeopaths
2 Artizan Road
Northampton NN1 4HU
Tel. 01604 21400

Traditional Acupuncture Society
1 The Ridgway
Stratford-upon-Avon
Warwickshire CV37 9JL
Tel. 01789 298798

Useful Addresses

AUSTRALIA

Hospitals
Repatriation Hospital
Daws Road
Daw Park
SA 5041
Tel. (08) 8276 9666

Royal Hobart Hospital
4 Illna Way
Blackmans Bay
TAS 7052
Tel. (03) 6229 3426

Royal Perth Hospital
Wellington Street
Perth
WA 6000
Tel. (09) 224 2186

Royal Prince Alfred Hospital
Missenden Road
Camperdown
Sydney
NSW 2050
Tel. (02) 9515 6111

St Vincent's Catholic Church Hospital
Darlinghurst
Sydney
NSW 2010
Tel. (02) 9332 7111

Townsville General Hospital
342 Stanley Street
Townsville
QLD 4810
Tel. 077 75 4141

Warrnambool and District Base Hospital
325 Timor Street
Warrnambool
VIC 3280
Tel. (03) 364 0625
Fax. (03) 364 0425

Support
The Hepatitis C Council
PO Box 432
Darlinghurst
Sydney
2010 NSW
Tel. (02) 9332 1599
Toll free: 1–800 803 990

CANADA

Information
The Canadian Liver Foundation
365 Bloor Street East, Suite 200
Toronto
Ontario M4W 3L4
Toll free: 1-800 563 5483

Support
The Hepatitis C Survivors Society (Canada)
c/o St Thomas Anglican Church
383 Huron Street
Toronto
Ontario M5S 2G5
Tel. (416) 979 5855
Toll free: 1-800 652 HEPC

IRELAND

Irish Haemophilia Society
4–5 Eustace Street
Temple Bar
Dublin 2
Ireland
Tel. 003531 677 8529

NEW ZEALAND

Hospital
The Liver Unit
Auckland Hospital
Park Road
Auckland
Tel. (09) 379 7440

Support
NZ Hepatitis C Support Group
Auckland Hospital
Private Bag 92024
Auckland
Toll free: 0800 22 4372

SOUTH AFRICA

Johannesburg General Hospital
Jubilee Street
Parktown
Johannesburg
Tel. 11 488 4911

UNITED STATES OF AMERICA

American Liver Foundation (ALF)
1425 Pompton Avenue
Cedar Grove
NJ 07009
Tel. 1-800-GO-LIVER
1-888-4-HEP-ABC
Website http://www.liverfoundation.org
Email info@liverfoundation.org

The ALF can supply information on how the problem of hepatitis is perceived and dealt with in America. Its quarterly publication, *Progress*, contains updates on new treatments.

Centers for Disease Control and Prevention
Hepatitis Branch, Mailstop G37
1600 Clifton Road, NE
Atlanta
GA 30333
Hepatitis hotline 404 332 4555
Public inquiries 1 800 311 3435

HCV Global Foundation
5337 College Ave.
PO Box 636
Oakland
CA 94618
Tel. 707 425 5343
Fax. 510 569 3743

Hepatitis Foundation International
30 Sunrise Terrace
Cedar Grove
NJ 07009
Tel. 1 800 891 0707
Website http://www.hepfi.org

Transplant Recipient International Organization
1735 Eye Street NW
Suite 917
Washington
DC 20006
Tel. 202 293 0980

Chronic Disease Self-Management Course
c/o Kate Lorig
Stanford University
Patient Education Research Center
1000 Welch Road, Suite 204
Palo Alto
CA 94304
Tel. 650 723 7935
Website http://www.stanford.edu/group/perc/perchome.html
Email Lorig@Leland.Stanford.edu

Index

Index